Internal Medicine Issues in Palliative Cancer Care

D0818304

Internal Medicine Issues in Palliative Cancer Care

Edited by

David Hui, MD, MSc

Assistant Professor of Palliative Care and Rehabilitation Medicine
Division of Cancer Medicine
The University of Texas MD Anderson Cancer Center
Houston, Texas

Eduardo Bruera, MD

Professor of Palliative Care and Rehabilitation Medicine
Division of Cancer Medicine
The University of Texas MD Anderson Cancer Center
Houston, Texas

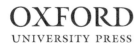

OXFORD
UNIVERSITY PRESS

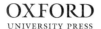

Oxford University Press is a department of the University of
Oxford. It furthers the University's objective of excellence in research,
scholarship, and education by publishing worldwide.

Oxford   New York
Auckland   Cape Town   Dar es Salaam   Hong Kong   Karachi
Kuala Lumpur   Madrid   Melbourne   Mexico City   Nairobi
New Delhi   Shanghai   Taipei   Toronto

With offices in
Argentina   Austria   Brazil   Chile   Czech Republic   France   Greece
Guatemala   Hungary   Italy   Japan   Poland   Portugal   Singapore
South Korea   Switzerland   Thailand   Turkey   Ukraine   Vietnam

Oxford is a registered trademark of Oxford University Press
in the UK and certain other countries.

Published in the United States of America by
Oxford University Press
198 Madison Avenue, New York, NY 10016

© Oxford University Press 2014

All rights reserved. No part of this publication may be reproduced, stored in
a retrieval system, or transmitted, in any form or by any means, without the prior
permission in writing of Oxford University Press, or as expressly permitted by law,
by license, or under terms agreed with the appropriate reproduction rights organization.
Inquiries concerning reproduction outside the scope of the above should be sent to the
Rights Department, Oxford University Press, at the address above.

You must not circulate this work in any other form
and you must impose this same condition on any acquirer.

Library of Congress Cataloging-in-Publication Data
Internal medicine issues in palliative cancer care / edited by David Hui, Eduardo Bruera.
    p. ; cm.
Includes bibliographical references and index.
ISBN 978–0–19–932975–5 (alk. paper)
I. Hui, David, 1975– editor of compilation.   II. Bruera, Eduardo, editor of compilation.
[DNLM: 1. Neoplasms—therapy.   2. Palliative Care—methods.   3. Comorbidity.
4. Hospice Care—methods.   5. Internal Medicine—methods.   QZ 266]
RC271.P33
616.99′4029—dc23   2013039278

This material is not intended to be, and should not be considered, a substitute for medical
or other professional advice. Treatment for the conditions described in this material is highly
dependent on the individual circumstances. And, while this material is designed to offer accurate
information with respect to the subject matter covered and to be current as of the time it was
written, research and knowledge about medical and health issues are constantly evolving and
dose schedules for medications are being revised continually, with new side effects recognized
and accounted for regularly. Readers must therefore always check the product information and
clinical procedures with the most up-to-date published product information and data sheets
provided by the manufacturers and the most recent codes of conduct and safety regulations. The
publisher and the authors make no representations or warranties to readers, express or implied,
as to the accuracy or completeness of this material. Without limiting the foregoing, the publisher
and the authors make no representations or warranties as to the accuracy or efficacy of the drug
dosages mentioned in the material. The authors and the publisher do not accept, and expressly
disclaim, any responsibility for any liability, loss, or risk that may be claimed or incurred as a
consequence of the use and/or application of any of the contents of this material.

9 8 7 6 5 4 3 2 1
Printed in the United States of America
on acid-free paper

Contents

Preface

Patients with advanced cancer often develop a number of clinical complications related to tumor progression and/or cancer treatments. In addition, the majority of these patients are elderly and they often have multiple comorbidities that require appropriate assessment and management. In the palliative stage of their disease, patients undergo a progressive transition from active acute care to community-based hospice care. This transition requires modification in the diagnostic tests, monitoring procedures, and pharmacologic treatments to adjust them to the palliative and short-term nature of the care.

The purpose of this book is to provide an update on the management of common clinical issues encountered in the delivery of palliative cancer care. Our main purpose is not to discuss specific palliative care assessments and management but to focus on the practical management of the main internal medicine issues as palliative care and hospice teams progressively become the primary care providers of patients.

This book is unique because it explains internal medicine through a prognosis-based framework, and provides a practical approach to maximizing comfort and quality of life while minimizing aggressive investigations and therapies for patients with life-limiting disease. Given that patients with advanced cancer often present with complex internal medicine problems, decision making regarding diagnostics and therapeutics requires a good understanding of state-of-the-art internal medicine and palliative care principles. It is the goal of this book to educate clinicians about these fundamental principles and to transform them into practical pearls for learners and practicing clinicians. This book is particularly relevant because palliative care is evolving from a predominantly community-based practice to the acute care setting, in which a good grasp of the complexities of various internal medicine issues is essential for care delivery.

This book includes 49 common internal medicine topics under various subspecialties. Our goal is to provide practical, succinct, evidence-based, and user friendly information for readers. It is primarily aimed at physicians, mid-level providers, nurses, pharmacists, and students involved in delivering palliative care to cancer patients in acute care facilities, inpatient hospices, nursing homes, or at home.

Although every effort has been made to ensure the accuracy of information in this handbook, the authors, editors, and publisher are not responsible for omissions, errors, or any consequences that result from application of the information contained herein. *Verification of the information in this manual is the professional responsibility of the clinician. Readers are strongly urged to consult other appropriate clinical resources prior to applying information in this manual, particularly medication dosages, for direct patient care.* This is particularly important since patterns of practice and clinical evidence evolve constantly. We welcome any constructive feedback to help make this manual a more accurate, practical, comprehensive, and user-friendly resource.

Editors
David Hui, MD, MSc
Eduardo Bruera, MD

Contributors

Zubia S. Ahmad, MD
Virginia Commonwealth University
    School of Medicine
VCU Massey Cancer Center
Richmond, Virginia

M. Cristina Ajenjo, MD
Department of Internal Medicine
Pontificia Universidad Catolica
    de Chile
Santiago, Chile

Robert M. Arnold, MD
Professor of Medicine
Division of General Internal Medicine
University of Pittsburgh
UPMC-Montefiore Hospital
Pittsburgh, Pennsylvania

Joseph Arthur, MD
Assistant Professor of Palliative Care
    and Rehabilitation Medicine
Division of Cancer Medicine
The University of Texas MD
    Anderson Cancer Center
Houston, Texas

Ahsan Azhar, MD
Division of Cancer Medicine
The University of Texas MD
    Anderson Cancer Center
Houston, Texas

**Ammar Chaudhary, MBChB,
ABIM, FRCPC**
University of British Columbia
St. Paul's Hospital
Vancouver, British Columbia
Canada

Shalini Dalal, MD
Associate Professor of Palliative Care
    and Rehabilitation Medicine
Division of Cancer Medicine
The University of Texas MD
    Anderson Cancer Center
Houston, Texas

Maxine de la Cruz, MD
Assistant Professor of Palliative Care
    and Rehabilitation Medicine
Division of Cancer Medicine
The University of Texas MD
    Anderson Cancer Center
Houston, Texas

Egidio Del Fabbro, MD
Associate Professor of
    Internal Medicine
Virginia Commonwealth University
    School of Medicine
VCU Massey Cancer Center
Richmond, Virginia

Marvin O. Delgado-Guay, MD
Assistant Professor of Palliative Care
    and Rehabilitation Medicine
Division of Cancer Medicine
The University of Texas MD
    Anderson Cancer Center
Houston, Texas

Rony Dev, DO
Assistant Professor of Palliative Care
    and Rehabilitation Medicine
Division of Cancer Medicine
The University of Texas MD
    Anderson Cancer Center
Houston, Texas

Daniel E. Epner, MD

Associate Professor of Palliative Care
and Rehabilitation Medicine
Division of Cancer Medicine
The University of Texas MD
Anderson Cancer Center
Houston, Texas

Marilene Filbet, MD

Unité de Soins Palliatifs
Centre Hospitalier de Lyon Sud
Hospices Civils de Lyon
Lyon, France

Susan Gaeta, MD

Assistant Professor of Critical Care
Division of Anesthesiology and
Critical Care
The University of Texas MD
Anderson Cancer Center
Houston, Texas

Caroline Ha, MD

Department of Internal Medicine
University of Texas Medical School
Memorial Hermann–Texas
Medical Center
Houston, Texas

Holly M. Holmes, MD

Assistant Professor Internal Medicine
Division of Internal Medicine
The University of Texas MD
Anderson Cancer Center
Houston, Texas

Kunal C. Kadakia, MD

Division of Internal Medicine
The University of Texas MD
Anderson Cancer Center
Houston, Texas

Kyung Ho Kim, MD, PhD

Hallym University College of Medicine
Kangdong Sacred Heart Hospital
Seoul, Korea

Gil Kimel, MD, FRCPC

Department of Medicine
University of British Columbia
St. Paul's Hospital
Vancouver, British Columbia
Canada

Meiko Kuriya, MD

Seirei Mikatahara Hospital
Shizuoka, Japan

Jung Hye Kwon, MD, PhD

Associate Professor of
Hematology-Oncology and
Internal Medicine
Hallym University College of
Medicine
Kangdong Sacred Heart Hospital
Seoul, Korea

Masanori Mori, MD

National Cancer Center
Tokyo, Japan

Linh Nguyen, MD

Assistant Professor of Geriatric and
Palliative Medicine
The University of Texas Health
Science Center at Houston
Medical School
Houston, Texas

Pedro Pérez-Cruz, MD, MPH

Programa Medicina Paliativa
Facultad de Medicina
Pontificia Universidad Catolica
de Chile
Santiago, Chile

Shobha Rao, MD

UT Physicians Hospice & Palliative
Medicine and Geriatric Medicine
University of Texas Medical School
Houston, Texas

Akhila Reddy, MD
Assistant Professor of Palliative Care
    and Rehabilitation Medicine
Division of Cancer Medicine
The University of Texas MD
    Anderson Cancer Center
Houston, Texas

Wadih Rhondali, MD, MSc
Unité de Soins Palliatifs
Centre Hospitalier de Lyon Sud
Hospices Civils de Lyon
Lyon, France

Jeffrey B. Rubins, MD
Director, HCMC Palliative Medicine
Department of Family Medicine and
    Community Health
University of Minnesota
Minneapolis, Minnesota

Jane O. Schell, MD
Assistant Professor of Medicine
University of Pittsburgh
UPMC-Montefiore Hospital
Pittsburgh, Pennsylvania

Beatriz Shand, MD, MBE
Instructor of Bioethics
Department of Neurology
Pontificia Universidad Catolica de Chile
Santiago, Chile

Robinder Singh, MD, FRCPC
Division of Cardiology
University of British Columbia
St. Paul's Hospital
Vancouver General Hospital
Vancouver, British Columbia
Canada

Kimberson Tanco, MD
Assistant Professor of Palliative Care
    and Rehabilitation Medicine
Division of Cancer Medicine
The University of Texas MD
    Anderson Cancer Center
Houston, Texas

**Mustafa Toma, MD, MS,
FRCPC ABIM**
Clinical Assistant Professor
Division of Cardiology
University of British Columbia
St. Paul's Hospital
Vancouver, British Columbia
Canada

Ivo W. Tremont-Lukats, MD
Assistant Professor of
    Neuro-Oncology
Division of Cancer Medicine
The University of Texas MD
    Anderson Cancer Center
Houston, Texas

Marieberta Vidal, MD
Assistant Professor of Palliative Care
    and Rehabilitation Medicine
Division of Cancer Medicine
The University of Texas MD
    Anderson Cancer Center
Houston, Texas

Paul Walker, MD
Associate Professor of Palliative Care
    and Rehabilitation Medicine
Division of Cancer Medicine
The University of Texas MD
    Anderson Cancer Center
Houston, Texas

Jenny Wei, DO
Department of Internal Medicine
University of Texas Medical School
Memorial Hermann–Texas
    Medical Center
Houston, Texas

**Donna S. Zhukovsky, MD,
FACP, FAAHPM**
Professor of Palliative Care and
    Rehabilitation Medicine
Division of Cancer Medicine
The University of Texas MD
    Anderson Cancer Center
Houston, Texas

Section I
Introduction

Chapter 1

Principles of Internal Medicine in Palliative Care

David Hui and Eduardo Bruera

Internal Medicine for Patients with Advanced Cancer

Cancer is one of the leading causes of mortality and morbidity, with one in three persons diagnosed with cancer in their lifetime. Cancer patients often have multiple comorbid diagnoses, such as chronic obstructive pulmonary disease (COPD), heart failure, and chronic kidney disease. These conditions may be a result of the neoplastic process, such as direct infiltration and obstruction. Alternatively, cancer treatments such as surgery, radiation, and systemic therapy can adversely affect organ function (e.g., anthracyclines and heart failure). Other comorbidities may be related to lifestyle choices (e.g., smoking and COPD). The remainder of conditions may be unrelated to or even predate the cancer diagnosis. Taken together, cancer and various comorbidities can contribute to significant symptom expression and psychological distress, resulting in a decreased quality of life and increased caregiver burden.

Management of cancer and these comorbidities may be even more complicated in patients with a short life expectancy. These patients typically have a poor performance status, a high symptom burden, and significant care needs, necessitating a unique approach to optimal care (Figure 1.1).

Decision Making in Medicine

Clinicians are confronted with a myriad of clinical decisions and ethical dilemmas on a daily basis. Proper management includes making sound decisions on both diagnosis and treatment. Which diagnostic test is the most appropriate? Is this therapy going to help or harm this patient? These decisions are often guided by a balance between the risks and benefits based on the existing clinical evidence. Although the literature is indispensable for providing the average risks and benefits, it is often difficult to apply these numbers to the individual patient. Furthermore, many clinical trials specifically exclude patients with a poor prognosis, and their findings may not apply to the palliative care population. Faced

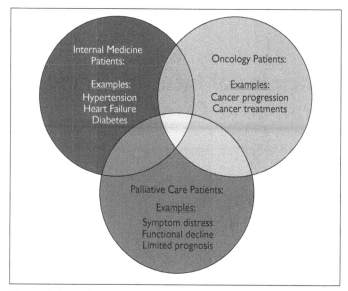

Figure 1.1 Overlap between internal medicine, oncology, and palliative care.

with these challenges, clinicians often need to tailor decisions to the individual patient based on multiple factors (Figure 1.2):

- Patient factors—Expected survival, performance status, comorbidities, preference, social factors, logistics, and social and family support are all crucial to clinical decision making.
- Disease factors—The curability of cancer, aggressiveness of disease, and mutation status can affect the choice of investigation/therapy. For aggressive disease in the adjuvant setting, more intensive regimens are indicated. For aggressive disease in the palliative setting, less aggressive therapy should be used.
- Clinician factors—The level of training, personal experience, and local healthcare resources are some key determinants of clinical decisions.

Decision-Making Styles

- The paternalistic (passive) approach involves the clinician deciding for the patient based on best clinical judgment.
- The autonomy (active) approach involves the clinician providing adequate information regarding the risks and benefits for patients to decide for themselves.
- A shared decision-making approach involves the clinician making a specific recommendation based on an explicit understanding of the patient's preference, while taking into consideration other important factors such as prognosis and comorbidities.

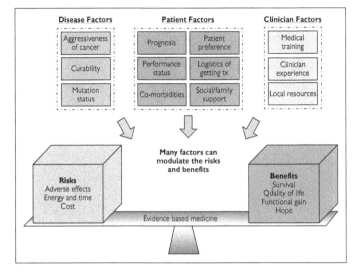

Figure 1.2 Medical decision making is based on the balance of risks and benefits.

Prognosis-Based Decision Making

Personalized medicine involves not only making treatment decisions based on the cancer's mutation status, but also providing recommendations tailored to the many other biological, psychosocial, logistical, and financial factors that are important to the patient. One of the most critical factors affecting clinical decision making is prognosis (Chapter 2). Specifically, the approach to clinical investigation and treatment for a patient with years of survival may be drastically different from that for a patient with only days or weeks to live (Figure 1.3). At the end of life (i.e., months or less of survival), a number of special considerations need to be taken into account in the decision-making process.

- In general, the risks of complications and adverse events with treatments increase significantly in patients at the end of life, while the potential benefits decrease dramatically. This shift in risk-to-benefit ratio favors a less aggressive approach.
- At the end of life, patients' goals of care may shift from life prolongation to comfort care.
- For patients with only weeks of survival, a 7-day hospital admission may take up a large proportion of the precise time remaining. Some patients may prefer to receive treatments at home even if they are not as effective (e.g., oral instead of intravenous antibiotics).
- Delirium at the end of life may complicate the patient's decision-making ability, symptom expression, and treatment choices.
- The difficulty in prognosticating accurately and the paucity of evidence in managing patients with a very poor prognosis make it challenging for clinicians to provide recommendations.

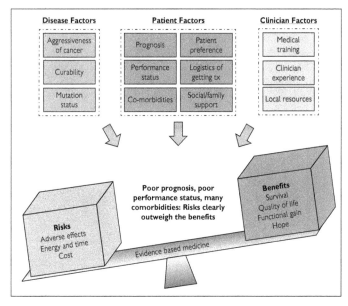

Disease Factors	Patient Factors		Clinician Factors
Aggressiveness of cancer	Prognosis	Patient preference	Medical training
Curability	Performance status	Logistics of getting tx	Clinician experience
Mutation status	Co-morbidities	Social/family support	Local resources

Poor prognosis, poor performance status, many comorbidities: Risks clearly outweigh the benefits

Benefits
Survival
Quality of life
Functional gain
Hope

Risks
Adverse effects
Energy and time
Cost

Evidence based medicine

Figure 1.3 The risks of treatment may outweigh the benefits for patients with a poor prognosis.

- These patients generally have significant comorbidities (e.g., pulmonary embolism, pneumonia) and decreased performance status, which could affect their ability to complete investigations and receive therapy.
- Investigations to confirm a suspected diagnosis without altering clinical management should be avoided at the end of life. Furthermore, patients may often be too frail to travel for tests and appointments.
- Medications used to prevent long-term complications may be unnecessary in patients with less than a few months to live. In contrast, treatments with a quick onset of action and symptom benefit are favored in these patients.
- Discharge decisions and place of care are often guided by how long a patient is expected to live.
- Symptomatic treatments may have a positive effect on the biomedical outcome (i.e., antibiotics for pneumonia). In other instances, symptomatic management could have a negative impact on the biomedical outcome (e.g., inotrope and heart failure, dexamethasone for dyspnea in a patient with pneumonia).

In summary, decision making regarding clinical investigations and treatments in the palliative care setting often requires special considerations. Clinicians caring for cancer patients with a poor prognosis need to master the principles of internal medicine, oncology, and palliative care, with particular attention paid to specific factors that could shift the balance between risks and benefits. This book aims to provide a concise review on the management of various internal medicine issues through the lens of oncology and palliative care.

Oncologists and Palliative Care Specialists Involvement in Managing the Internal Medicine Issues

This book is designed for clinicians working in the fields of primary care, oncology, and palliative care. It provides the basics of prognosis-based management of common internal medicine issues in cancer patients and is not intended to replace the need for primary care or specialty involvement. One practical question is how much of the internal medicine issues should the oncologists and/ or palliative care specialists address? For instance, should the oncology team, palliative care team, and/or medicine team be involved in treating a patient with advanced lung cancer who is admitted with pneumonia and COPD exacerbation? How about stable heart failure in a cancer patient with metastatic pancreatic cancer currently receiving home hospice care? This depends on multiple factors, including:

- Patient factors
  - Complexity of the medical issue(s)—Patients with highly complex medical issues requiring frequent monitoring and treatment adjustments are best managed by specialists familiar with the issues.
  - Patient preference—Patients who have a long-standing relationship with their primary care physician and specialists may want to continue follow-up at their offices. Other patients who are bed bound may choose to receive all of their care from the hospice team.
- Clinician factors
  - Knowledge and expertise—Each clinician should identify his or her own level of comfort in managing the general medical issues.
  - Time—The amount of time is a key determinant of how much one can deliver. Teams that are skilled may be able to deliver care more efficiently.
- Logistical issues
  - Healthcare setting—The attending team is often responsible for addressing the concurrent medical issues for hospitalized patients, and may involve other specialists if the need arises. Hospice patients often receive much of their care through the hospice team.
  - Institutional policy and clinical resources—Local policy and the availability of resources such as staffing and supplies may guide the level of involvement.

In summary, the roles of oncologist, palliative care specialist, primary care clinicians, and other specialists may evolve depending on the ever-changing patient factors, clinician factors, and logistical factors. The key is to ensure good communication with patients, their caregivers, and other healthcare professionals to streamline care delivery and to formulate an individualized management plan.

Recommended Reading

1. Hui D. *Approach to Internal Medicine (3rd ed.)*. Springer, New York, 2010.
2. El Osta B, Bruera E. Models of Palliative Care Delivery. In Bruera E, Higginson IJ, Ripamonti C, von Gunten C (eds.). *Textbook of Palliative Medicine (2nd ed.)*. Hodder Arnold, London, 2006: 266–276.

Chapter 2

Principles of Prognostication

David Hui

Prognostication Is Essential for Decision Making

- Personal decision making for patients
  - Healthcare decisions—Patients who are aware of their poor prognosis are less likely to choose chemotherapy and other aggressive measures at the end of life.
  - Personal decisions—Saying goodbye to my loved ones, selling stocks, going on a vacation, starting legacy projects.
  - Advance care planning—Establishment of a will, funeral plans, healthcare proxy, power of attorney, and an out-of-hospital do-not-attempt resuscitate order—is partly based on the understanding of a limited prognosis. These decisions may also evolve over time depending on the trajectory of the illness. It is also important for patients to make plans for their place of care and to know how they can get help with activities of daily living and instrumental activities of daily living when their function declines.
- Medical decision making for clinicians
  - Investigations such as blood work or imaging may be withheld if a patient has only days of life expectancy.
  - Systemic cancer therapy use in the last 14 days of life is considered an indicator of poor end-of-life care.
  - Major interventions such as total parenteral nutrition, gastrostomy, and dialysis are contraindicated in patients with only a few weeks of survival.
  - Hospice referral is based on a prognosis of 6 months or less.
  - Antidepressants often take weeks before patients experience any benefits, and thus are not helpful in patients with days of prognosis.
  - Medications for hyperlipidemia may have a limited role in patients with only a few months to live.

Estimating Survival in Patients with Advanced Cancer (Foreseeing)

- Clinician prediction of survival
  - Temporal question—"How long will this patient live?" The prognostic accuracy with this approach is 20–30%.
  - Surprise question—"Would you be surprised if this patient died in 1 week?" The accuracy is up to 90%.
  - Probabilistic question—"What is the probability this patient will be alive in 1 week?" The accuracy of this approach is between 60% and 90%.

Table 2.1 Palliative Prognostic Score (PaP Score)

Prognostic Factor	Score
Dyspnea	1
Anorexia	1.5
Karnofsky performance status 40% or less	2.5
Clinician prediction of survival	
11–12 weeks	2
7–10 weeks	2.5
5–6 weeks	4.5
3–4 weeks	6
1–2 weeks	8.5
Total white blood cell count	
8,500–11,000/mm^3	0.5
>11,000/mm^3	1.5
Lymphocyte percentage	
12–19.9%	1
0–11.9%	2.5
Interpretation of total score	**Median survival/30 day survival**
0–5.5	76 days/87%
5.6–11	32 days/52%
11.1–17.5	14 days/17%

- Prognostic factors
  - Clinical—Poor performance status, dyspnea, anorexia-cachexia, delirium.
  - Laboratory—Elevated C-reactive protein, leukocytosis, lymphopenia, elevated lactate dehydrogenase, hypoalbuminemia, hypercalcemia.
- Prognostic models
  - Palliative prognostic score (see Table 2.1)—Combination of six prognostic factors.
  - Palliative prognostic index (see Table 2.2)—Combination of five prognostic factors.

Signs of Impending Death

- Presence of any of the following signs in patients with advanced cancer suggests that survival is likely in terms of days:
  - Palliative performance status ≤20%.
  - General appearance changes—Hyperextension of the neck, drooping of the nasolabial fold (decrease in prominence/visibility of the nasolabial fold), inability to close the eyelids.
  - Respiratory signs—Respiration with mandibular movement, death rattle (gurgling sound produced on inspiration and/or expiration related to airway secretions), grunting of vocal cords (sound produced predominantly on expiration, related to vibrations of the vocal cords), Cheyne–Stokes breathing, periods of apnea.

Table 2.2 Palliative Prognostic Index (PPI)	
Prognostic Factor	**Score**
Dyspnea at rest	3.5
Oral intake	
Moderately reduced	1
Severely reduced	2.5
Palliative performance status	
30–50%	2.5
10–20%	4
Edema	1
Delirium (not caused solely by a single medication)	4
Interpretation of total score	**Median survival (95% confidence interval)**
0–4	68 days (52–115 days)
5–6	21 days (13–33 days)
7–15	5 days (3–11 days)

- Cardiovascular changes—Pulselessness of the radial artery, peripheral cyanosis, mottling.
- Neurocognitive changes—Decreased responsiveness to verbal/visual stimuli, nonreactive pupils.

Communicating Survival (Foreseeing, "SPIKES")

- Setting
  - Find a quiet room for discussion.
  - Ideally sit down, talk to the patient at eye level, speak clearly and slowly.
  - Ask patients if they want their family to be present as well.
- Perception
  - What does the patient understand about his or her illness?
  - What has the patient been told about future treatments?
- Information
  - How is the prognostic information going to help?
- Knowledge
  - Acknowledge uncertainty in prognostication.
  - Provide prognosis in terms of general time frames (i.e., "years," "months," "weeks," "days") instead of median survival or vague terms ("not very good").
- Emotions
  - Respond to emotions appropriately.
  - Silence can sometimes be helpful.
  - Provide empathic responses such as "This is a difficult time for you." or "You have really gone through a lot already."

- Strategy
  - Communicate nonabandonment.
  - Ensure patient has a good follow-up plan (e.g., return visits). Make appropriate referrals to other services bases on the patient's needs (e.g., social work, psychology).
  - Every prognostic discussion is an opportunity to empower the patient and to discuss advance care planning.

Relevance to the Cancer Palliative Care Setting

- A majority of cancer patients want to know their prognosis. They also want their physicians to communicate with them in an honest and compassionate manner.
- Prognostic discussion should be a longitudinal process. It begins at the time of cancer diagnosis and continues with changes in health status, such as the initiation of new systemic therapy due to disease progression, hospital admissions, abrupt decline in performance status, or when the patient is clearly dying.

Recommended Reading

1. Glare PA, Sinclair CT. Palliative medicine review: prognostication. *J Palliat Med* 2008;11(1):84–103.
2. Hui D, Kilgore K, Nguyen L, Hall S, Fajardo J, Cox-Miller TP, Palla SL, Rhondali W, Kang JH, Kim SH, Del Fabbro E, Zhukovsky DS, Reddy S, Elsayem A, Dalal S, Dev R, Walker P, Yennu S, Reddy A, Bruera E. The accuracy of probabilistic versus temporal clinician prediction of survival for patients with advanced cancer: a preliminary report. *J Palliat Med* 2012;15(8):902–909.
3. Baile WF, Buckman R, Lenzi R, Glober G, Beale EA, Kudelka AP. SPIKES–A six-step protocol for delivering bad news: application to the patient with cancer. *Oncologist* 2000;5(4):302–311.

Chapter 3

Principles of Advance Care Planning

Donna S. Zhukovsky

What Is Advance Care Planning (ACP) and Why Does It Matter?

- ACP reflects an *ongoing* process of communication among patients, families, and other loved ones, surrogate decision makers, and healthcare providers where prognostic information, therapeutic options, and patient's life goals, values, and wishes for further treatment are understood and addressed to better honor patient preferences.
- ACP allows individuals to plan for future healthcare in the event of decisional incapacity.
- ACP may be conducted with healthy individuals and may begin anywhere along the cancer continuum including patients who have newly diagnosed cancer, potentially curable cancer, relapsed cancer, metastatic cancer, progressive cancer, or cancer in remission with prolonged survivorship.
- Effective ACP facilitates selection of optimal medical and nonmedical care options throughout the disease trajectory, including patients who retain their capacity for medical decision making, as well as those who do not.
- ACP does NOT typically result in increased distress for patients or surrogate decision makers and is associated with fewer bereavement complications for surrogate decision makers.

Key Components of Advance Care Planning

- Predicated on expert communication among the individual, his or her surrogate decision maker, and clinicians, meaningful ACP is an example of patient-centered care and requires (Figure 3.1):
  - Understanding, reflecting, and discussing the individual's health state and care options in the context of his or her values and goals.
  - Formulating and documenting a plan.
  - Communicating the plan to involved loved ones and the medical team.
  - Reviewing the plan periodically to ensure that it remains consistent with values and goals, especially with changes in health conditions.
  - Enacting the plan under the appropriate circumstances.

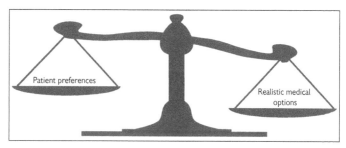

Figure 3.1 Advance care planning involves longitudinal discussions between the patients and clinicians to find a balance between patient preferences and realistic medical options.

- Most patients prefer that ACP:
  - Take place in the outpatient setting.
  - Occur in a period of relative health stability.
  - Be initiated by their physician.

Communication of Advance Care Plans and Advance Directives

- Communication of advance care plans occurs as part of the ACP process when key stake holders are involved:
  - The patient
  - His or her surrogate decision maker
  - Family and other loved ones
  - Involved clinicians
- Accessibility of advance care plans to the healthcare team is supported by completion of advance directives that are transparent and are easily available to the healthcare team.
- Advance directives may
  - Be instructional (i.e., living will).
  - Specify a surrogate decision maker for periods of incapacity for medical decision making (i.e., medical power of attorney, durable power of attorney for healthcare, healthcare proxy).
  - Convert patient preferences into physician orders (i.e., out of hospital do not resuscitate order forms [OOH DNR], medical orders for life-sustaining therapy [MOLST], physician orders for life-sustaining therapy [POLST]).
- Instructional documents and forms converting patient preferences into order forms indicate the patient's preferences for *or* against certain types of treatments—they do not universally signal that patients request withholding or withdrawing treatments. For example, they may include orders indicating that transfer to the intensive care unit is acceptable, but the individual does not want cardiopulmonary resuscitation (CPR) or they may state not to transfer the patient to the hospital and no CPR.

- Advance directives may be statutory or advisory in nature:
  - Statutory documents are based on legal requirements codified in state law. Many states will honor statutory documents from other states.
  - Advisory documents are not codified in state law, but carry legal weight if they provide clear evidence of the patient's wishes.
  - Statutory forms for instructional documents and those that designate a surrogate decision maker are not available in all states.
- If a patient does not have the capacity for medical decision making and does not have an advance directive that specifies a surrogate decision maker, one will be selected from a legal hierarchy that varies from state to state.
  - For patients who are separated but still married, the surrogate decision maker is typically the spouse and for those who are estranged from their family, the appointed individual may be someone who is not familiar with their values and goals and may not have their best interests at heart.

Clinician Role in Supporting Meaningful ACP

- Systematically incorporate ACP into patient care.
- Introduce the topic in the outpatient setting during a period of stability, whenever possible.
- Clarify that you would like to understand his or her concerns and what is important to them in the event that complications arise in order to support medical decision making that is congruent with the patient's values and goals.
- Encourage the patient to bring his or her surrogate decision maker to the appointment so that they may also better understand the patient's values and goals for future healthcare.
- Ascertain the patient and family's understanding of the disease process and prognosis and available treatment options and clarify inconsistencies.
- Do NOT start the process by talking about withholding or withdrawing treatments, as this is not the goal of the ACP process. By ensuring that key stakeholders are on the same page with understanding of the medical situation and care options and that the patient's values and goals have been identified, preferences for and against available care options follow more easily.
- Ensure transparency of the advance care plan and the availability of advance directives in all care settings (i.e., home, office, hospital, assisted living facility, nursing home).
- Revisit the care plan periodically, especially with changes in the individual's health status, to ascertain its consistency with current values and goals for healthcare.
- When discussing the choice of a surrogate decision maker with the patient:
  - Emphasize the selection of an agent who is familiar with the person's values and goals for healthcare.
  - Confirm the willingness of the proposed surrogate decision maker to accept the responsibility of the role.
  - Involve the surrogate decision maker in advance care planning discussions.

- Ascertain the surrogate's ability to make decisions based on the patient's wishes and not his or her own personal wishes.
- Clarify the degree of flexibility the patient grants the surrogate decision maker in the decision-making process and let the surrogate decision maker know the choice. Do they want that person to follow their stated preferences precisely or do they allow them discretion to deviate from previously articulated preferences based on what they think would be best at the time?

Advance Care Planning for Patients with Years of Life Expectancy

- For these patients, introducing the concept of ACP, helping them consider values and goals for decision making in general scenarios (i.e., if their ability to recognize people or think was lost) and focusing on the selection of a surrogate decision maker may be sufficient.

Advance Care Planning for Patients with Months of Life Expectancy

- As these patients have experience with the disease process, expand the above discussions to include prognosis and possible complications that may arise to help patients think through their options in more specific scenarios. These preferences can then be documented in the form of a living will and medical power of attorney or similar document. Care choices here may be medical and nonmedical, including preferred place of death, care of children/guardianship, financial and emotional support of loved ones, and legacy-making activities. Care choices may also be documented in the form of physician orders.

Advance Care Planning for Patients with Weeks/Days of Life Expectancy

- With this group of patients, it is important to add discussions about desired spiritual practices and activities, funeral plans, and memorial services.

Relevance to the Cancer Palliative Care Setting

- Patients with cancer experience many care choices, complications, and stressors throughout the cancer experience. By thoughtful facilitation of meaningful advance care planning, clinicians can offer their patients and families more control over a devastating situation, with care choices that are congruent with the individual's values and goals. This, in turn, leads to decreased stress for patients, families, and the healthcare team, with less conflict at times of crisis.

Recommended Reading

1. Fins JJ, Maltby BS, Friedmann E, et al. Contracts, covenants and advance care planning: an empirical study of the moral obligations of patient and proxy. *J Pain Symptom Manage* 2005;29(1):55–68.

2. Sudore RL, Fried TR. Redefining the "planning" in advance care planning: preparing for end-of-life decision making. *Ann Intern Med* 2010;153(4):256–261.

3. Wendler D, Rid A. Systematic review: the effect on surrogates of making treatment decisions for others. *Ann Intern Med* 2011;154(5):336–346.

4. Zhukovsky DS, Bruera E. A transcultural perspective of advanced directives in palliative care. In *Palliative Medicine,* Chapter 109. Edward Arnold Ltd., London, 2006: 1035–1043.

Section II

Pulmonary

Chapter 4

Chronic Obstructive Pulmonary Disease

Jeffrey B. Rubins

Description

- Chronic obstructive pulmonary disease (COPD) is characterized by incompletely reversible airflow limitation that usually is progressive, is caused by an abnormal pulmonary inflammatory response to noxious exposures, and is associated with significant extrapulmonary effects. Typical noxious exposures are inhaled tobacco smoke, smoke from biomass fuels, and environmental particulates.

Symptoms and Signs

- Pulmonary symptoms diagnostic of disease—Shortness of breath (especially with exertion and at night), cough (typically productive of sputum), and exacerbations (flares of disease requiring intensification of treatment and that are associated with increased COPD mortality).
- Additional systemic symptoms—Anxiety, depression, social isolation, psychological distress, poor sleep, fatigue, anorexia, constipation.
- Signs—Usually not present until the disease has progressed to at least moderate airflow obstruction; include hyperinflated chest, use of accessory muscles of respiration, wheezing or decreased breath sounds, and a prolonged expiratory phase.

Investigations

- Spirometry—Required for diagnosis [based on the ratio of forced expiratory volume in 1 second (FEV_1) to forced vital capacity (FVC) <0.70, and assessment of severity (based on FEV_1 as percent predicted].
- Pulse oximetry—If chronically ≤88% indicates the need for supplemental oxygen to prolong survival.
- Arterial blood gases—In addition to assessing for hypoxemia, they are used to determine the degree of hypoventilation.

Relevance to the Cancer Palliative Care Setting

• COPD is a life-limiting and prevalent chronic disease in adults, particularly among patients with tobacco-related cancers. Patients with COPD have many palliative needs, including more debilitating dyspnea and worse physical limitation than seen in cancer alone, with a high proportion of patients becoming house bound and socially isolated.

Management of Patients with Years of Life Expectancy

• Recommendations for management of all COPD patients (Table 4.1):
  • If still smoking, counsel and assist with tobacco cessation.
  • Inoculate annually with influenza vaccine and once with pneumococcal vaccine (revaccinate according to Centers for Disease Control guidelines).
  • Enroll in pulmonary rehabilitation program.
  • Prescribe short-acting bronchodilators as needed.
  • Recommendations for management of more severe COPD patients:
  • More severe disease is indicated by worse spirometry (FEV$_1$ <50% predicted), worse symptoms (dyspnea caused by lesser amounts of exertion), and more frequent exacerbations (two or more during the previous year).
  • Add inhaled long-acting bronchodilators—Either a long-acting anticholinergic agent or a combination of an inhaled long-acting β-agonist and inhaled corticosteroids.
  • Provide continuous supplemental home oxygen if the resting oxygen saturation during the stable state is ≤88%.
  • Treat exacerbations with a 2-week course of systemic steroids, a course of antibiotics if sputum has become more purulent, and more frequent use of short-acting bronchodilators.

Management of Patients with Months of Life Expectancy

• Relief of refractory dyspnea:
  • Dyspnea refractory to the treatments for airflow obstruction can be relieved by the addition of long-acting opioids and the use of a fan blowing air on the face.
  • When studied, supplemental oxygen has **not** been proven to relieve dyspnea except for hypoxemic patients and should not be obligatory for patients who do not perceive benefit.
  • Noninvasive positive pressure ventilation (commonly but improperly called "BIPAP") can be useful during sleep and as needed during the day to relieve dyspnea in some patients, but may be poorly tolerated and should not be forced upon patients who do not perceive any benefit.

Table 4.1 Typical Pharmacologic Therapy for Stable COPD in the United States

Class	Common Medications and Doses
Short-acting antichlolinergics	Ipratropium bromide MDI two puffs (40 µg) inhaled four times a day
	Ipratropium bromide solution 2.5 mL (0.5 mg) by nebulizer inhaled four times a day
Long-acting anticholinergics	Tiotropium bromide DPI one capsule (18 µg) inhaled once per day
Short-acting β_2-agonists	Albuterol sulfate MDI two puffs (200 µg) inhaled every 4 to 6 hours as needed
	Albuterol sulfate solution 3 mL (2.5 mg) by nebulizer inhaled every 4 to 6 hours as needed
	Levalbuterol tartrate MDI two puffs (90 µg) inhaled every 4 to 6 hours as needed*
	Levalbuterol HCl solution 0.63 mg by nebulizer inhaled every 6 to 8 hours as needed*
Long-acting β_2-agonists	Formoterol fumarate DPI one capsule (12 µg) inhaled every 12 hours
	Formoterol fumarate solution one vial (20 µg) by nebulizer inhaled every 12 hours
	Salmeterol xinafoate DPI one inhalation (50 µg) every 12 hours
	Arformoterol tartrate solution one vial (15 µg) by nebulizer every 12 hours
	Indacaterol DPI one capsule (75 µg) inhaled once a day
Combination short-acting β_2-agonists and antichlolinergics	Albuterol plus ipratropium bromide MDI two puffs (180 µg/35 µg) inhaled four times a day
	Albuterol plus ipratropium bromide solution 3 mL (2.5 mg/0.5 mg) by nebulizer four to six times per day
Inhaled corticosteroids	Beclomethasone dipropionate 80–160 µg inhaled twice a day*
	Budesonide DPI 400–800 µg inhaled twice a day*
	Budesonide solution 0.5 mg by nebulizer inhaled twice a day*
	Fluticasone MDI 88–220 µg inhaled twice a day*
	Mometasone furoate DPI 440 µg inhaled twice a day*
Combination products	Salmeterol/fluticasone propionate DPI (50 µg/250 µg) one inhalation twice a day
	Budesonide/formoterol fumarate dihydrate DPI (160 µg/4.5 µg) one inhalation twice a day
	Fluticasone furoate/vilanterol DPI (100 µg/25 µg) one inhalation daily
Methylxanthines	Theophylline sustained-release tablet 100–600 mg orally per day (adjusted to serum level of 8–12 µg/mL)
Phosphodiesterase-4-inhibitors	Roflumilast tablet 500 µg orally per day

*Not FDA approved for treatment of COPD.
MDI, metered-dose inhaler; DPI, dry-powder inhaler.

- Tobacco cessation at this point in the disease is unlikely to improve survival and may cause transient worsening of respiratory secretions and increased dyspnea. Influenza and pneumococcal vaccinations are similarly unlikely to improve survival.

- Advance directives regarding ventilator support—COPD patients are at high risk for respiratory failure, which may require prolonged and possibly chronic invasive ventilation. The trajectory of COPD, with its insidious onset, gradual progression of disease, and episodic worsening followed by recovery back to "normal" life, leads many afflicted patients to see COPD more as a way of life to be accepted rather than as a life-limiting disease. Some may even have already required invasive ventilation during an exacerbation and were successfully extubated and discharged from the hospital. As a result, COPD patients are often disinclined to consider limitation of life-sustaining treatments. Supportive discussions regarding end of life wishes, including the possibility of time-limited trials of invasive ventilation with defined stopping points, can prevent undesired deaths on chronic ventilator support.

Management of Patients with Weeks/Days of Life Expectancy

- Systemic opioids, the use of fans, and medications to relieve anxiety become the mainstay of therapy.

- As patients lose their ability to use inhalers effectively, bronchodilators can be converted to nebulized formulations, if these are tolerated and relieve symptoms.

- Systemic steroids should be continued while patients are able to take medications orally.

- Antibiotics may be used to palliate cough and shortness of breath if caused by purulent secretions.

Recommended Reading

1. The Global Strategy for the Diagnosis, Management and Prevention of COPD, Global Initiative for Chronic Obstructive Lung Disease (GOLD), 2013. Available at http://www.goldcopd.org/.

2. Disler RT, Currow DC, Phillips JL, Smith T, Johnson MJ, Davidson PM. Interventions to support a palliative care approach in patients with chronic obstructive pulmonary disease: an integrative review. *Int J Nurs Studies* 2012;49(11):1443–1458.

3. Heigener DF, Rabe KF. Palliative care concepts in respiratory disease. *Respiration* 2011;82(6):483–491.

Chapter 5

Pleural Effusion

Jeffrey B. Rubins

Classification/Causes

- Pleural effusions related to underlying cancer
  - Malignant effusions—Most common in lung and breast cancer, lymphoma (both Hodgkin's and non-Hodgkin's), mesothelioma, colon cancer, and ovarian cancer. Malignant effusions indicate a very poor prognosis in such patients, with a median survival of 4 months.
  - Paramalignant effusions
    - Indirect effects of the cancer—Most commonly (1) parapneumonic effusions in pneumonia, caused by depressed immune defenses and/or by endobronchial obstruction; (2) effusions from pulmonary embolism, related to hypercoaguability from increased levels of tissue factor or activation of the coagulation cascade; (3) cylothorax from obstruction of the thoracic duct by involved mediastinal nodes; (4) transudative effusions by obstruction of the superior vena cava.
    - Effects of treatment
      - Radiation-induced—Chest irradiation for lung cancer, mesothelioma, lymphoma, or breast cancer can cause a direct radiation pleuritis resulting in pleural effusion (usually appearing within 6 months of treatment). Also, mediastinal irradiation can produce mediastinal fibrosis, which in turn can produce chylous effusions by obstruction of pleural lymphatic drainage.
      - Drug-induced—Chemotherapy can produce pleuritis and pleural effusions, most commonly with the use of methotrexate, procarbazine, cyclophosphamide, bleomycin, docetaxel, imatinib, and dasatinib.
- Pleural effusions unrelated to underlying cancer—Typically indicate systemic disease, and the history, examination, and investigation are directed toward the diagnosis of these underlying diseases.

Symptoms and Signs

- Symptoms—Shortness of breath, pleuritic pain, cough, hiccups (rarely).
- Signs—Tachypnea, dullness to percussion, and decreased breath sounds on the affected side.

Investigations

- The extent and invasiveness of the diagnostic evaluation will depend upon the presence of symptoms, the size and rate of recurrence of the effusion, the performance status and prognosis of the patient, and whether metastatic cancer has already been diagnosed.
- Chest imaging [radiography and computed tomography (CT)]—Necessary to confirm the presence and size of the effusion; it also provides important information including the presence of parenchymal disease (infiltrates, masses), loculations, endobronchial obstruction, pleural thickening, and shift of the mediastinum (which if toward the side of the effusion suggests trapped lung).
- Chest ultrasound—Useful to guide thoracentesis. May also detect nodules or masses in the pleural space, which strongly indicate malignant involvement, and may be needle-biopsied with ultrasound guidance.
- Thoracentesis
  - Diagnostic—Indicated for the initial evaluation of any cancer patient with an unexplained pleural effusion large enough to safely aspirate (more than 10 mm in depth on a lateral decubitus film), and for recurrent idiopathic effusions prior to diagnostic thoracoscopy, if planned. Commonly performed under ultrasound guidance when available, especially if the effusions are small or loculated, or if the patient is at higher risk of complications from the procedure.
  - Therapeutic—Indicated for patients with shortness of breath. Although typically as much fluid as possible is removed, draining even 300 mL of fluid is sufficient to determine whether reducing pleural pressures will relieve dyspnea. Generally, up to 1,500 mL of fluid can be removed without concern for reexpansion pulmonary edema. However, in patients with trapped lung, far less fluid can be safely removed, and thoracentesis should always be stopped whenever the patient reports increasing chest pain or shortness of breath.
  - Laboratory studies—Fluid should be sent for chemistry [lactate dehydrogenase (LDH), protein] to classify the effusion as transudate or exudate, for cultures, and (at least 60 mL) for cytology.
  - Relief of symptoms—Should always be assessed and documented after therapeutic thoracentesis to guide further management; many cancer patients do not have relief of symptoms, either because the underlying lung cannot reexpand or because the dyspnea is caused by other underlying conditions.
  - Postprocedure imaging—A chest radiograph should be obtained immediately after thoracentesis to determine to what degree the lung has reexpanded, and to establish a baseline for comparison with future films to determine if the effusion recurs. The presence of a hydropneumothorax on the postprocedure film, especially when the apparent volume of airspace within the lung appears unchanged, signals a trapped lung. Chest CT may be useful in such situations to image the thickness of the pleura and determine the best treatment strategy. Chest CT with angiography

may also be helpful if the lung has reexpanded but the patient reports no relief of dyspnea, and to evaluate for lymphangitic carcinomatosis, thromboembolism, tumor embolism, and other nonmalignant cardiopulmonary diseases that can produce dyspnea.

- Surgical or medical thoracoscopy—Thoracoscopic pleural biopsy has diagnostic yields up to 95% for malignant effusions and is indicated for undiagnosed exudative effusion after thoracentesis with negative cytology when proof of malignant pleural effusion will alter management. Surgical biopsy by video-assisted thoracoscopy (VATS) allows better inspection and biopsy of the parietal pleura but is contraindicated if the patient's medical condition is too tenuous to tolerate the general anesthesia and single-lung ventilation required for the procedure. Where available, medical thoracoscopy can be performed under conscious sedation and local anesthesia in an endoscopy suite but often yields smaller pleural biopsies than those obtained by VATS.

Relevance to the Cancer Palliative Care Setting

- Pleural effusions in cancer patients may indicate metastatic malignancy, infection, or thromboembolism, or may be related to underlying systemic diseases.
- When symptomatic, palliative therapies should be chosen based upon maximizing the patient's quality of life. Repeated serial thoracentesis, pleurodesis, or placement of indwelling tunneled catheters are palliative options to consider, depending upon prognosis and patient choices.

Management of Patients with Years of Life Expectancy

- Cancer patients with small asymptomatic pleural effusions for whom diagnosing a malignant effusion will not change management do not need intervention other than observation.
- For cancer patients with symptomatic pleural effusions, the goals are to provide relief of dyspnea, minimize discomfort, and limit hospitalization time.
- Patients with effusions due to small cell lung cancer, and for some with effusions from lymphoma and germ-cell tumors, may have relief of effusions and symptoms from chemotherapy. For other cancer patients with better performance status (Karnofsky score of 70 or higher) whose lung reexpands after the initial thoracentesis and who have relief of dyspnea, pleurodesis should be considered for recurrence of a symptomatic effusion.
- Pleurodesis typically requires admission to the hospital for drainage of the effusion and sclerosis and is most commonly done by placement of a pleural catheter and instillation of talc slurry, or by insufflation of talc powder using medical thoracoscopy or VATS. The main disadvantage of pleurodesis by pleural catheter or chest tube is that a longer hospitalization may be required to fully drain the effusion prior to instillation of the sclerosing agent, but

this approach avoids the need for general anesthesia and intubation, typically used when pleurodesis is performed using VATS. Where available, medical thoracoscopy has emerged as an intermediate option to quickly explore the pleural surfaces, drain the effusion, and insufflate talc powder for pleurodesis under conscious sedation without requiring intubation.

Management of Patients with Months of Life Expectancy

- For cancer patients with poor performance status (Karnofsky score <70) and/or months of life expectancy, recurring symptomatic pleural effusions can be managed with repeated outpatient thoracentesis, which avoids hospitalization for more invasive and potentially morbid procedures.
- However, when symptomatic effusions are recurring quickly, insertion of an indwelling tunneled catheter is an increasingly used option. The catheter can be inserted as an outpatient procedure, and the effusion can be drained at home or nursing facility as frequently as necessary to relieve symptoms. Although this avoids hospitalization, it transfers care of the catheter and drainage of the effusion to the patient and caregivers. Indwelling pleural catheters have been shown to be equivalent or better than pleurodesis for relief of dyspnea and improvement in quality of life and can induce spontaneous pleurodesis in 25–50% of patients within 1–2 months after placement. However, approximately 20% of patients have complications related to the catheter (chest pain, catheter obstruction, local cellulitis, tumor seeding of the catheter track, and pleural infection).

Management of Patients with Weeks/Days of Life Expectancy

- Symptoms of dyspnea, pain, and cough from pleural effusions are most appropriately managed with medications.
- For patients with indwelling pleural catheters, drainage of fluid can be done as frequently as necessary, as long as this provides relief of symptoms and does not itself cause discomfort.

Recommended Reading

1. Doelken P. Management of pleural effusion in the cancer patient. *Semin Respir Crit Care Med* 2010;31:734–742.

2. Rodriguez-Panadero F, Romero-Romero B. Management of malignant pleural effusions. *Curr Opin Pulmon Med* 2011;17(4):269–273.

3. Rubins JB. Pleural effusion. *Medscape* 2012 June 21. Available at http://emedicine.medscape.com/article/299959-overview.

Chapter 6

Pulmonary Embolism

Marieberta Vidal

Classification

- Acute—Symptoms develop immediately after obstruction of pulmonary vessel.
- Chronic—Might be asymptomatic or can develop progressive dyspnea due to pulmonary hypertension.
- Massive—Causes hypotension or other catastrophic events that usually result in right ventricular failure or death.
- Submassive—Pulmonary embolism (PE) that does not meet the criteria for massive PE.

Symptoms and Signs

- Symptoms—Dyspnea, pleuritic pain, cough, orthopnea, and wheezing. In acute PE, the onset of dyspnea is usually seconds to minutes.
- Signs—Tachypnea, tachycardia, hypoxemia, hypotension, decreased breath sounds, rales, an accentuated pulmonic component of the second heart sound, pleural friction rub, pleural effusion, jugular venous distension, and low-grade fever.

Investigations

- Angiography—"Gold standard" in the diagnosis of acute PE. It is an invasive procedure but is generally considered safe and well tolerated in the absence of hemodynamic instability.
- Spiral CT—Spiral (helical) computed tomography (CT) scanning with intravenous contrast. It can also help to detect other pulmonary conditions.
- V/Q scan—Diagnostic accuracy is greatest when it is combined with clinical probability. A normal test excludes PE. Useful for patients with allergies, iodinated contrast, or impaired renal function.
- D-Dimer—Good sensitivity and negative predictive value, but poor specificity and positive predictive value. Levels >500 ng/mL are considered abnormal.

Relevance to Cancer Palliative Care Settings

- Patients with advanced cancer are at higher risk of developing a PE.
- Deep vein thrombosis (DVT) of the upper extremities can also contribute to PE.
- Symptomatic PE can significantly affect the quality of life of cancer patients who develop dyspnea and pain.

Management for Patients with Years of Life Expectancy

- Pulmonary embolism has a mortality rate of approximately 30% if untreated. The clinical presentation can range from asymptomatic to cardiopulmonary shock.
- Hemodynamic support and oxygen should be started if the patient presents with hypotension and hypoxemia.
- If there is a high clinical suspicion for pulmonary embolism and no clear contraindications, empiric anticoagulation should be started as soon as possible.
- Thrombolytic therapy can be used after confirmed diagnosis of PE has been established in patients with hemodynamic compromise. Because of the increased risk of bleeding, the risks and benefits should be carefully evaluated.
- In patients with hemodynamic compromise but in whom thrombolytic therapy is contraindicated or failed, embolectomy is an option.
- Intravenous unfractionated heparin is the preferred agent after thrombolysis and the initial therapy for all patients who do not have severe circulatory failure.
- Low-molecular-weight heparin (LMWH) is recommended for hemodynamically stable cancer patients. In severely obese patients, consider antifactor Xa testing to avoid overdosing or underdosing. Antifactor Xa testing is also recommended in patients with severe renal insufficiency because of the increased risk of bleeding. Unfractionated heparin is preferred in renal patients (Table 6.1).
- In the absence of hypoxemia, serious comorbidities, high risk of bleeding, and abnormal vital signs, patients can usually be treated in the ambulatory setting.

Management for Patients with Months of Life Expectancy

- Management is similar to patients with years of life expectancy.

Management of Patients with Weeks/Days of Life Expectancy

- There is limited evidence about the treatment of pulmonary embolism at the end of life.

Table 6.1 Pharmacologic Therapy for Acute Pulmonary Embolism

Class	Common Medications and Doses
Low-molecular-weight heparin	Dalteparin 200 units/kg subcutaneously once a day for 30 days, then 150 units/kg daily
	Enoxaparin 1 mg/kg subcutaneously twice per day or enoxaparin 1.5 mg/kg daily
	Nadroparin 171 units/kg subcutaneously daily
	Tinzaparin 175 units/kg subcutaneously daily
Unfractionated Heparin	Unfractionated heparin 80 units/kg load, then 18 units/kg per hour intravenously to target activated partial thromboplastin time (aPTT) of 2–2.5× control
Fondaparinux	Fondaparinux 5 mg (<50 kg), 7.5 mg (50–100 kg), or 10 mg (>100 kg) subcutaneously daily

- The focus of treatment is symptom control and comfort. This can usually be achieved by opioids and supplemental oxygen (if hypoxemic) in patients with significant dyspnea.
- At the end of life, patients might develop acute renal insufficiency that could complicate the use of LMWH.
- Frequent blood work or injections should be avoided.
- Patients' goals of care and preferences should be considered.

Recommended Reading

1. Kearon C, Akl EA, Comerota AJ, et al. Antithrombotic therapy for VTE disease: Antithrombotic Therapy and Prevention of Thrombosis, 9th ed: American College of Chest Physicians Evidence-Based Clinical Practice Guidelines. *Chest* 2012;141:e419S.

2. Noble SI, Shelley MD, Coles B, et al. Management of venous thromboembolism in patients with advanced cancer: a systematic review and meta-analysis. *Lancet Oncol* 2008;9:577.

3. Djulbegovic B. Management of venous thromboembolism in cancer: a brief review of risk-benefit approaches and guidelines' recommendations. *J Support Oncol* 2010;8:84.

4. Farge D, Debourdeau P, Beckers M, et al. International clinical practice guidelines for the treatment and prophylaxis of venous thromboembolism in patients with cancer. *J Thromb Haemost* 2013;11:56.

Chapter 7

Noninvasive Ventilation

Susan Gaeta

Indications

Noninvasive ventilation (NIV) can be used for the treatment of acute respiratory failure depending on the etiology.
- Respiratory failure
  - Hypercapnic chronic obstructive pulmonary disease (COPD) exacerbation
  - Cardiogenic acute pulmonary edema
  - Postoperative acute respiratory failure
  - Patients with immune deficiencies
  - Hypoxemic respiratory failure (unclear benefit)
- Dyspnea relief
  - Especially if hypercapnic respiratory failure

Contraindications

- Patients who are not alert enough to protect their airway or who have increased secretions failure.
- Patients with recent upper airway or gastrointestinal surgery.

Investigations

- Chest x-ray to evaluate for pneumonia or pulmonary edema.
- Computed tomography (CT) scan of chest may be considered to assist in determining the potential etiology of respiratory failure.
- Arterial blood gas to assist with adjustment of NIV.

Relevance to the Cancer Palliative Care Setting

- Cancer patients often have comorbid conditions that may need to be treated simultaneously to assist with symptom burden.
- Use of NIV in the appropriate patient may improve survival and quality of life by potentially reducing the need for endotracheal intubation and the risk of ventilator-associated infections.

- Use of NIV may allow patients to be able to communicate with their families and potentially remain in the palliative care unit or ward depending on hospital policy.

Management for Patients with Years of Life Expectancy

- Commencement of NIV for potentially reversible causes of acute respiratory failure but goals of care should to be discussed in regard to the need to consider endotracheal intubation if there is no improvement with NIV.
- It is important to treat the underlying causes:
  - Steroids and bronchodilators for COPD exacerbation and consider antibiotics as appropriate.
  - Diuretics for treatment of acute cardiogenic pulmonary edema.
- Anxiolytics may be needed to treat anxiety due to the use of NIV.
- May need to be transferred to the ICU based on the support required by NIV and if the plan is to proceed to endotracheal intubation.
- NIV can be considered in patients who failed extubation, particularly in patients with COPD or congestive heart failure (CHF). These patients need to be monitored closely.

Management for Patients with Months of Life Expectancy

- Management is similar to patients with years of life expectancy. In addition, review of the goals of care and prognosis need to be discussed with the patient and the patient's family in regard to considering the inappropriateness of endotracheal intubation based on the overall prognosis.

Management for Patients with Weeks/Days of Life Expectancy

- Management is similar to patients with months of life expectancy; however, it is also recommended that comfort care measures be considered and not commence NIV.
- Delirium and decreased level of consciousness are common in the last days of life, and may be relative contraindications to NIV.

Recommended Reading

1. Azoulay E, Demoule A. Palliative noninvasive ventilation in patients with acute respiratory failure. *Intensive Care Med* 2011;37:1250–1257.
2. Keenan SP, Tasnim T. Clinical practice guidelines for the use of noninvasive positive-pressure ventilation and noninvasive continuous positive airway pressure in the acute care setting. *CMAJ* 2011;83(3):E195–214.

Section III

Cardiovascular

Chapter 8

Heart Failure

Ammar Chaudhary and Gil Kimel

Classifications

- Heart failure (HF) with reduced ejection fraction (EF) or HF with preserved EF (~50% prevalence)
- Left-sided, right-sided, or biventricular failure
- Acute, chronic, or acute on chronic HF
- Low-output or high-output failure
- Dilated, hypertrophic, or restrictive cardiomyopathy
- Warm (normal perfusion) and dry (euvolemic), warm and wet, cool and dry, cool and wet

Etiology

- Coronary artery disease
- Hypertension
- Valvular—Functional, degenerative, myxomatous, infectious, rheumatic, autoimmune, congenital, carcinoid, radiation, congenital, anorexic agents, iatrogenic
- Myocardial
  - Myocarditis—Infectious [Coxsackie, adenovirus, parvovirus B19, HIV, hepatitis C, cytomegalovirus, herpes simplex virus (HSV), Epstein–Barr virus (EBV), Chagas' disease], autoimmune [systemic lupus erythematosus (SLE), dermatomyositis, rheumatoid arthritis (RA), scleroderma], idiopathic (giant cell, lymphocytic)
  - Toxins—Alcohol, heavy metals, drugs (anthracyclines, trastuzumab, cocaine)
  - Genetic—Hypertrophic, familial dilated, arrythmogenic right ventricular cardiomyopathy (ARVC), left ventricular (LV) noncompaction, ion channelopathies [long QT, Brugada, short QT, catecholaminergic polymorphic ventricular tachycardia (CPVT)], neuromuscular, mitochondrial
  - Infiltrative/storage—Amyloidosis, sarcoidosis, hemochromatosis, liposomal storage disease (Fabry's, Gaucher's), mucopolysaccharidosis (Hurler's, Hunter's)
  - Others: Tachycardia-mediated, stress-induced "tako-tsubu," peripartum, endocrine [diabetes, thyroid (amiodarone toxicity), pheochromocytoma],

endomyocardial fibrosis, hypereosinophilic syndromes, idiopathic dilated (20–30%)

- Pericardial—Effusion with tamponade [malignancy, viral infection, post-myocardial infarction (MI), autoimmune, uremia, hypothyroidism], constriction (radiation, prior surgery, recurrent pericarditis)

Precipitants

- Decompensation of chronic HF (lack of compliance with dietary restrictions or medications), ischemia, hypertension, infections (commonly pneumonia), arrhythmia, anemia, pulmonary embolism, renal dysfunction

Symptoms and Signs

- Symptoms—Dyspnea (New York Heart Association class I–IV), paroxysmal nocturnal dyspnea, orthopnea, lethargy, abdominal distension, peripheral edema, dizziness, weight gain, or cardiac cachexia
  - NYHA Class I—No symptoms (shortness of breath) with ordinary physical activity.
  - NYHA Class II—Mild symptoms during ordinary activity.
  - NYHA Class III—Symptoms during less-than-ordinary activity.
  - NYHA Class IV—Symptoms while at rest.
- Signs—Hypotension (reduced cardiac output and medications) or hypertension (when HF is precipitated by hypertension), pulsus paradoxus (tamponade), tachycardia, tachypnea, reduced level of consciousness (LOC), cyanosis, cool peripheries, elevated jugular venous pressure (JVP), displaced apex, S3, systolic murmur of functional mitral regurgitation, pulmonary edema, pleural effusion, ascites, hepatomegaly, sacral and lower limb edema

Investigations

- Brain natriuretic peptide (BNP)—HF is likely when the BNP is >400 pg/ml, possible when the BNP is between 100 and 400 pg/ml, and unlikely when the BNP is <100 pg/ml.
- Complete blood count (CBC), electrolytes, and creatinine [estimated glomerular filtration rate (eGFR)] may help identify HF precipitants (anemia, infection), renal dysfunction due to drug therapy or the cardiorenal syndrome, and electrolyte disturbances.
- An electrocardiogram (ECG) can determine precipitants such as arrhythmia (e.g., atrial fibrillation) or ischemia. Voltages are reduced in pericardial effusion and infiltrative cardiomyopathies. QTc prolongation is common with drugs (e.g., antiemetics). The presence of isolated right or bilateral pleural

effusions is common. Noncardiac causes of dyspnea (e.g., pneumonia) can also be evaluated.

- Echocardiography is used for the assessment of biventricular systolic and LV diastolic function, LV geometry, valves, and the pericardium.
- Cardiac magnetic resonance imaging (MRI) is superior in assessing biventricular systolic function and enables the evaluation of the myocardium for causes of cardiomyopathies and viability.

Relevance to the Cancer and Palliative Care Setting

- HF may occur as a result of cancer treatments such as anthracyclines (early or late), previous chest radiation, and targeted agents such as trastuzumab. Close monitoring of cardiac function is needed when patients are on these treatments.
- HF may contribute to symptom burden and can cause significant fatigue and dyspnea. In patients with these symptoms and a reasonable life expectancy, screening for HF may be warranted.

Management of Patients with Years of Life Expectancy

- Lifestyle modifications include fluid (<1.5 L/day) and salt (<2 g/day of Na) restriction. When appropriate, patients should be advised to weigh themselves and titrate diuretics accordingly.
- Medication—Diuretics are the mainstay for symptom management, although loop diuretics may be ineffective in reducing malignancy-induced edema. Opioids have been shown to relieve dyspnea due to pulmonary edema (Table 8.1).
- The following treatments may be appropriate in patients who have an expected prognosis estimated as months to years.
  - LV dysfunction requires afterload reduction with angiotensin-converting enzyme (ACE) inhibitors [or angiotensin receptor blockers (ARBs) for patients intolerant of ACE inhibitors and hydralazine and nitrates for those with significant renal dysfunction].
  - β-Blockers should be instituted when patients are near euvolemia and uptitrated to achieve maximally tolerated target doses (HR 60). Discontinuation of β-blockers should be done with caution as patients may experience palpitations or anxiety. We generally recommend continuation of β-blockers even as the patient nears end of life.
  - Spironolactone (or epleronone, especially in intolerant patients due to gynecomastia) is indicated when the NYHA II and EF are < 30% (or EF 30–35% and QRS > 130 ms).
  - Inotropes have not been shown to improve survival, but they can be helpful short-term for dyspnea management in decompensated HF.

Table 8.1 Pharmacologic Therapy for Heart Failure

Class	Name	Initial Dose	Target Dose
ACE inhibitors	Captopril	12.5 mg TID	25–50 mg TID
	Enalapril	2.5 mg BID	10 mg BID
	Lisinopril	2.5 mg daily	20 mg daily
	Perindopril	2 mg daily	8 mg daily
	Ramipril	1.25–2.5 mg BID	5–10 mg BID
	Trandolapril	1 mg daily	4 mg daily
Angiotensive receptor blockers	Candesartan	4 mg daily	32 mg daily
	Valsartan	40 mg BID	160 mg BID
β-Blockers	Bisoprolol	1.25–2.5 mg daily	10 mg daily
	Carvedilol	3.125 mg BID	25–50 mg BID
	Metoprolol tartrate	12.5 mg BID	100 mg BID
	Metoprolol succinate	100 mg daily	200 mg daily
Mineralocorticoid antagonists	Spironolactone	12.5 mg daily	50 mg daily
	Eplerenone	25 mg daily	50 mg daily
Loop diuretics	Furosemide	20 mg BID	120 mg BID
	Bumetanide	0.5 mg BID	4 mg BID
	Torsemide	10 mg daily	200 mg daily
	Ethacrynic acid	50 mg daily	200 mg daily
Thiazide diuretics	Hydrochlorothiazide	25 mg daily	100 mg daily
	Metolazone	2.5 mg daily	10 mg BID

- Treatment of diastolic HF is limited to symptom and risk factor management [i.e., diuretics and control of hypertension (HTN)].
- Device therapy with an implantable cardiac defibrillator (ICD) for prevention of sudden cardiac death is indicated in patients with an EF ≤ 35%, if NYHA II or III, 40 days post-MI, or in NYHA I if the EF is ≤ 30%. Patients with non-ischemic cardiomyopathy should be considered for an implantable cardiac defibrillator (ICD) if NYHA II or III and EF ≤ 35% or if NYHA I and EF are ≤ 35% (weak recommendation). Cardiac resynchronization therapy (CRT) reduces morbidity and mortality if NYHA II, the EF is <30% (or < 35% if NYHA III–IV), and the QRS >120 ms. Patients with advanced malignancy are generally not good candidates for new device therapy. Left ventricular assist devices (LVADs) and cardiac transplantations are options for end-stage HF, provided that the patient is cancer free for 5 years.

Management of Patients with Months of Life Expectancy

- Patients with an expected survival <1 year are generally precluded from ICD implantation.

- Patients who already have an ICD implanted should ordinarily have high-voltage shocking function deactivated; pacemaker and CRT functions are generally not deactivated.

Management for Patients with Weeks/Days of Life Expectancy

- At the end of life, patients may be treated with opioids and possibly diuretics for symptom management. Common symptoms include dyspnea, chest pain, and anxiety.
- Discontinuation of statin therapy is recommended.
- Continuation of β-blockers, antiarrhythmics, anticoagulants, and ACE inhibitors is recommended even as patients near end of life as if they are discontinued, symptoms (i.e., palpitations in the case of β-blockers) may worsen.
- Use of all other cardiac agents should be minimized to limit side effects and medication burden.
- Deactivation of ICDs is done by wirelessly reprogramming the device and does not require surgical removal of the device. In emergency situations, a magnet can be placed over the ICD, which deactivates the high-voltage shocking feature but does not deactivate the pacemaker function of the ICD.
- The focus of care must be on quality of life rather than prolongation of life.

Recommended Reading

1. Nohria A, Tsang SW, Fang JC, et al. Clinical assessment identifies hemodynamic profiles that predict outcomes in patients admitted with heart failure. *J Am Coll Cardiol* 2003;41:1797–1804.

2. Bonow RO, et al. *Braunwald's Heart Disease: A Textbook of Cardiovascular Medicine* (9th ed.). Saunders, Maryland Heights, MO, 2012.

3. ACC/AHA/HRS 2008 guidelines for device-based therapy of cardiac rhythm abnormalities: a report of the American College of Cardiology/American Heart Association Task Force on Practice Guidelines. *J Am Coll Cardiol* 2008;51:e1–62.

4. Singal PK, Iliskovic N. Doxorubicin-induced cardiomyopathy. *N Engl J Med* 1998;339:900–905.

Chapter 9

Acute Coronary Syndrome

Robinder Singh, Mustafa Toma, and Gil Kimel

Classification

Acute coronary syndrome (ACS) encompasses a spectrum of coronary artery disease (CAD), ranging from threatened to complete coronary occlusion, as well as manifestations of systematic disease (anemia, sepsis, etc.) resulting in myocardial ischemia/infarction.

- Unstable angina/non-ST elevation MI (UA/NSTEMI)—Syndrome of a new or worsening pattern of typical, exertional chest discomfort; possible electrocardiographic (ECG) changes and/or elevated biomarkers [troponin, creatinine kinase (CK)]. It represents a threatened or partial coronary occlusion.
- ST elevation MI (STEMI)—Symptoms and biomarker elevations are as above with the presence of ST elevation or new left bundle branch block (LBBB). Represents a complete coronary occlusion.

Symptoms and Signs

- Symptoms—Chest or left arm pain, radiation to right arm, radiation to both arms, radiation to neck. Classically, worsened by exertion and emotion and relieved with rest and nitroglycerin. Other symptoms include nausea and vomiting, shortness of breath, and palpitations.
- Signs—Third heart sound, hypotension, pulmonary crackles, diaphoresis, tachycardia, tachypnea, elevated jugular venous pulsation (JVP), fourth heart sound, murmur associated with mechanical complication (papillary muscle dysfunction/rupture, ventricular septal defect, lateral wall rupture), peripheral edema, and cool extremities (associated with shock state).

Investigations

- Blood work—Complete blood count, electrolytes, renal function (urea, creatinine), liver function tests, troponin (on presentation, q6h subsequently), CK, international normalized ratio (INR), activated prothrombin time (aPTT). Other blood work includes fasting glucose and lipid panel and hemoglobin A1C (Hb$_{A1C}$).
- Imaging—Chest x-ray (CXR), coronary CT angiogram, echocardiogram, myocardial perfusion imaging (for diagnosis, or to assess myocardium at risk/prognosis).

- ECG—New ST elevation, new Q-wave, any ST elevation, new conduction defect, new ST depression, any Q-wave, any ST depression, T-wave peaking/inversion, new T-wave inversion, any conduction defect.
- Coronary angiogram

Relevance to the Cancer Palliative Care Setting

- Risk factors such as smoking and advanced age are common to cancer patients and may place many patients at higher risk for concomitant CAD.
- Coronary intimal injury and fibrosis as a result of radiotherapy have been well documented as a cause of CAD in cancer patients (lymphomas, breast, lung, esophageal cancer).
- Chemotherapeutic agents (5-fluorouracil, capcetibine, bleomycin, estramustine) have been found to increase the risk of ACS in patients with underlying cancer. The mechanisms are unclear and may involve vasospasm.
- Patients are at increased risk of thrombosis and embolism from a variety of causes [nonbacterial thrombotic endocarditis (NBTE), disseminated intravascular coagulation (DIC)].
- Myocardial ischemia may occur in the setting of extreme stress, such as the initial diagnosis of cancer, severe anemia, sepsis, or other systemic manifestations/consequences of underlying malignancy. This is commonly referred to as "demand ischemia" and may not derive the same benefit from traditional therapy for ACS, although current data are sparse. Management of patients with demand ischemia should be tailored to the clinical situation.

Management of Patients with Years of Life Expectancy

- See Tables 9.1 and 9.2 for details of the management of ACS.

Table 9.1 Management of Acute Coronary Syndrome

Medication	Indications	Contraindications/Cautions	Comments
Nitroglycerin	Ongoing ischemic CP	Hypotension Concurrent use of PDE inhibitors	May be used even in end-stage disease
Anticoagulation (UFH, LMWH, fondaparinux)	All patients with ACS unless nearing end of life	Ongoing or high risk of bleeding History of HIT LMWH should not be used in those with eGFR<30 ml/min or age >75 years	

(continued)

Table 9.2 Continued

CHAPTER 9 Acute Coronary Syndrome

Medication	Indications	Contraindications/Cautions	Comments
Thrombolysis	Patients presenting with STEMI in a non-PCI capable center if presenting within 12 h of symptom onset Especially for those presenting within 3 h of symptom onset or with ongoing CP	Any prior ICH History of intracranial malignancy/AVM CVA within 3 months Active bleeding or bleeding diathesis Suspected aortic dissection	Not generally used in patients nearing end of life
PCI	Patients presenting with STEMI	Patients with ongoing bleeding or at high risk of bleeding on DAPT Patients with significant renal dysfunction Inability to lie flat	Can be used as a palliative procedure in patients with ongoing pain
ASA	All patients with ACS	Ongoing or high risk of bleeding (history of GI bleed, severe thrombocytopenia, etc.)	
P2Y$_{12}$ receptor inhibitors	All patients with ACS Especially in those treated with PCI	Ongoing or high risk of bleeding (history of GI bleeding, severe thrombocytopenia)	Not generally used in patients nearing end of life
ACE inhibitors/ARB	All patients with ACS Especially in the setting of anterior MI or with significant LV dysfunction	Hypotension Acute renal dysfunction Hyperkalemia	Generally continued even in patients nearing end of life
β-Blockers	All patients with ACS Especially in those with significant atrial/ventricular arrhythmias or with significant LV dysfunction	Hypotension/bradycardia Severe uncontrolled reactive airway disease Decompensated CHF/cardiogenic shock	Generally continued even in patients nearing end of life
Statins	All patients with ACS	Caution in patients with known liver dysfunction	Not generally continued in patients with end-stage heart disease
Mineralocorticoid receptor antagonists	Patients with MI complicated by significant LV dysfunction (LVEF <40%)	Significant renal dysfunction (eGFR <30) Hyperkalemia	

Abbreviations: ACS, acute coronary syndrome; ASA, acetylsalicylic acid; CHF, congestive heart failure; CP, chest pain; DAPT, dual antiplatelet therapy; eGFR, estimated glomerular filtration rate; GI, gastrointestinal; HIT, heparin-induced thrombocytopenia; LMWH, low-molecular-weight heparin; LV, left ventricular; LVEF, left ventricular ejection fraction; PDE, phosphodiesterase; STEMI, ST elevation myocardial infarction; UFH, unfractionated heparin.

Table 9.2 Common Medications in Acute Coronary Syndrome

Class	Doses
Acute Management	
Nitroglycerin	0.5 mg SL q5min ×3 acutely for angina 0.4 mg/h transdermal patch Nitro drip 25 mg in 250 ml D$_5$W, start at 5 µg/min IV, then ↑ by 5–10 µg/min every 3–5 min to 20 µg/min, then ↑ by 10 µg/min every 3–5 minutes up to 200 µg/min
Opioids	Morphine 2–5 mg SC q4h regular and q1h PRN Hydromorphone 1 mg SC q4h regular and q1h PRN
Anticoagulation	
Unfractionated heparin	50–70 U/kg IV bolus followed by 18 U/kg/h IV infusion to be adjusted to 1.5–2.5× normal aPTT
Low-molecular-weight heparin	30 mg IV bolus, then 1 mg/kg SC BID for at least 48 h and up to 8 days; is preferred in those undergoing no IV bolus for NSTEMI (caution if renal failure or age >75)
Fondaparinux	2.5 mg SC daily until discharge or 8 days
Antiplatelets	
ASA	162–325 mg PO load, then 81 mg daily indefinitely
P2Y$_{12}$ receptor inhibitors	Clopidogrel 300 mg PO load followed by 75 mg PO daily. Continued for a minimum of 2 weeks in the setting of thrombolytic therapy or conservative management Continued for a minimum of 1 month in the setting of PCI with bare metal stent (BMS) Continued for a minimum of 1 year in the setting of PCI with drug eluting stent (DES) Prasugrel To be used in the setting of PCI only 60 mg PO load, followed by 10 mg PO daily 1 month duration for BMS, 1 year for DES Ticegralor To be used in the setting of PCI only 180 mg PO load, followed by 90 mg PO BID 1 month duration for BMS, 1 year for DES
Adjunctive therapy	
ACE inhibitors	Enalapril_2.5 mg PO daily, titrated to 20 mg PO BID Captopril 6.25 mg PO TID, titrated to 50 mg PO TID Lisinopril 2.5–5 mg PO to start, titrate to 10 mg Ramipril 2.5 mg PO BID to start, titrate to 5 mg PO BID Trandolapril 0.5 mg PO daily to start, titrate to 4 mg PO daily
ARBs	Valsartan 20 mg PO BID, titrated to 160 mg PO BID
β-Blockers	Atenolol 50 mg PO daily to start, titrated to 100 mg PO daily Bisoprolol 10 mg PO daily Carvedilol 6.25 mg PO BID to start, titrated to 25 mg PO BID Metoprolol 12.5 mg PO BID to start, titrated to 50 mg PO BID

(continued)

Table 9.2 Continued	
Class	Doses
Mineralocorticoid receptor inhibitors	Eplerenone 25 mg PO daily to start, titrate to 50 mg PO daily
Statins	Atorvastatin 80 mg PO qHS (lower doses may be used in intolerant patients)
	Pravastatin 40 mg PO qHS

Management of Patients with Months of Life Expectancy

- Antiplatelets and anticoagulation may be reasonable if there is no increased risk of bleeding.
- Nitrates, β-blockade, and angiotensin-converting enzyme (ACE) inhibitors/ angiotensin receptor blockers (ARBs) may be initiated as antianginal therapy. Statins would not be beneficial.

Management of Patients with Weeks/Days of Life Expectancy

- Antianginals and opioids would be the only mainstay therapy. Transdermal, subcutaneous, or intravenous opioids and nitrates should be administered to patients who are unable to take oral medications.

Recommended Reading

1. Panju AA, et al. Is this patient having a myocardial infarction? *JAMA* 1998;280(14):1256–1263.

2. Anderson JL, et al. ACC/AHA 2007 guidelines for the management of patients with unstable angina/non-ST-elevation myocardial infarction. *Circulation* 2007;116:e148–e304.

3. Jneid H, et al. 2012 ACCF/AHA focused update of the guideline for the management of patients with unstable angina/non–ST-elevation myocardial infarction. *Circulation* 2011;123: e426–e579.

4. O'Gara PT, et al. 2013 ACCF/AHA guideline for the management of ST-elevation myocardial infarction. *Circulation* 2013;127:e362–e425.

5. Hui D. *Acute Coronary Syndrome in Approach to Internal Medicine (3rd ed.).* Springer, New York, 2010.

Chapter 10

Pericardial Disease

Robinder Singh, Mustafa Toma, and Gil Kimel

Classification

- Acute pericarditis—Pericardial inflammation from a variety of etiologies (see Table 10.1).
- Recurrent pericarditis—Recurrent inflammation, within days to weeks of cessation of therapy.
- Cardiac tamponade—Restriction of diastolic filling secondary to significant pericardial effusion or local compression (thrombus, mass).
- Constrictive pericarditis—Chronic inflammation leading to contraction and fibrosis of the pericardium and subsequent left and/or right heart failure (HF). It may develop after cardiac surgery, pericarditis, or radiation.

Table 10.1 Etiology of Percarditis	
Categories	Etiology
Cardiac	Aortic dissection, post-myocardial infarction (MI), cardiac surgery (Dressler's syndrome)
Drug induced	Anticoagulants, dantrolene, isoniazid, penicillin, thrombolytics, phenytoin, phenylbutazone, doxorubicin, procainamide, hydralazine
Iatrogenic	Catheter/pacemaker procedures, cardiopulmonary resuscitation (CPR)
Infectious	Viral, bacterial, fungal, mycoplasma, parasitic
Inflammatory	Behcet's disease, giant cell arteritis, granulomatosis with polyangiitis, mixed connective disease, lupus, rheumatoid arthritis, rheumatic fever, scleroderma, vasculitis, polyarteritis nodosa, sarcoidosis, inflammatory bowel disease (Crohn's, ulcerative colitis), Whipple's disease
Metabolic	Thyroid disease, uremia
Malignant	Lung or breast cancer, Hodgkin's disease, leukemia, melanoma, rhabdomyosarcoma, teratoma, fibroma, lipoma, leiomyoma, angioma
Radiation induced	Usually caused by radiotherapy treatment for chest malignancy
Traumatic	Sharp/penetrating injury, blunt force trauma

Symptoms and Signs

- Acute/recurrent pericarditis
  - Symptoms—Characteristic chest pain (acute onset, pleuritic, decreased with sitting up and leaning forward)
  - Signs—Fever, pericardial friction rub
- Cardiac tamponade
  - Symptoms—Dyspnea, fever, chest pain, cough
  - Signs—Tachycardia, pulsus paradoxus >10 mmHg, decreased heart sounds, hypotension, hypertension, tachypnea, pedal edema, pericardial rub, hepatomegaly, Kussmaul's sign
- Constrictive pericarditis
  - Symptoms—Dyspnea, orthopnea, palpitations, fatigue, edema, gastrointestinal symptoms
  - Signs—Elevated jugular venous pulsation (JVP) (Kussmaul's sign, prominent Y-descent), quiet heart sounds, pericardial knock, hepatosplenomegaly, ascites, edema

Investigations

- Labs—Complete blood count (CBC), electrolytes, renal function, liver enzymes, international normalized time (INR), activated partial thromboplastin time (aPTT), creatine kinase (CK), troponin. Consider erythrocyte sedimentation rate (ESR), C-reactive protein (CRP), antinuclear antibody (ANA), thyroid-stimulating hormone (TSH), HIV serology, and purified protein derivative (PPD) in appropriate clinical scenarios.
- Electrocardiogram (ECG)—Should be performed in all patients with suspected pericardial disease.
  - Acute pericarditis—Sinus tachycardia, diffuse concave ST elevation, PR depression
  - Cardiac tamponade—Low voltages, QRS alternans
- Imaging—Chest radiograph, echocardiogram, computed tomography/magnetic resonance imaging (CT/MRI)
- Invasive diagnostics—Right heart catheterization (constriction)
- Pericardiocentesis—Diagnostic and therapeutic benefits (tamponade). Fluid analysis includes pH, cell count and differential, Gram stain, culture, cytology, and acid-fast bacilli.

Relevance to the Cancer Palliative Care Setting

- Pericardial disease can occur as a direct result of malignancy or as a consequence of treatment, as is seen with radiation therapy and certain chemotherapeutic agents.

Management in Patients with Years of Life Expectancy

- Acute/Recurrent pericarditis—High-dose acetylsalicylic acid (ASA) (see Table 10.2) or nonsteroidal antiinflammatory drugs (NSAIDs) should be used as first-line therapy for acute pericarditis. Treatment should be reinitiated for a total of 4–8 weeks for recurrence. Colchicine should be added for adjuvant treatment and long-term prophylaxis for both acute (if not resolved with ASA or NSAIDS) and recurrent pericarditis. Prednisone may be used for connective tissue-mediated disease or in those with contraindications to ASA or NSAIDs, although there may be a high rate of recurrence and side effects. Surgical pericardectomy is rarely required; however, it can be considered in appropriate surgical candidates who have failed traditional medical therapy.

- Pericardial effusion/tamponade—Patients with symptomatic hypotension should be managed acutely with fluid resuscitation.
  - Pericardiocentesis—Should be performed in all symptomatic patients and in asymptomatic patients in whom the etiology of effusion is in question. Isolated pericardiocentesis in the setting of known, malignant pericardial effusion is generally not recommended, unless there is a very limited life expectancy (up to 60% recurrence rate).
  - Percutaneous drainage—Should be considered for patients at high risk of recurrence. Should be discontinued if output is less than 30–40 mL per day.
  - Balloon pericardiotomy—Can be considered in all patients at the time of initial pericardiocentesis, especially if there is a high likelihood of recurrence. May be considered as an alternative to surgical pericardiotomy in those with significant symptomatic reaccumulation.
  - Pericardial sclerosis—Sclerosing agents include tetracycline, doxycycline, minocycline, bleomycin, and talc. These agents can cause extreme pain when instilling into the pericardial space and have not been shown to have significant benefit as compared to traditional catheter drainage. This practice is thus outdated.
  - Surgical pericardiotomy—May be considered in appropriate candidates. A minimally invasive, video-assisted thoracoscopy (VATS) pericardiotomy would be recommended over the open surgical procedure.

- Constrictive pericarditis—Symptoms including dyspnea and edema may be managed with loop diuretics. Definitive management involves pericardiectomy in appropriate surgical candidates.

Table 10.2 Medical Management of Acute/Recurrent Pericarditis	
Class	**Common Medications/Doses**
ASA	650 mg PO TID/QID continued for 3–4 weeks, followed by slow taper
NSAIDs	Ibuprofen: 400–800 mg PO TID continued for days to weeks, can consider taper
	Indomethacin: 50 mg PO TID for 1–2 weeks, followed by slow taper
Colchicine	0.6 mg PO BID continued for 3 months
Prednisone	0.25–0.5 mg/kg/day for 2 weeks, followed by slow taper
Abbreviations: ASA, acetylsalicylic acid; NSAIDs, nonsteroidal antiinflammatory drugs.	

Management of Patients with Months of Life Expectancy

- Medical management—Should be initiated in patients with acute/recurrent pericarditis as outlined above (see Table 10.2).
- Invasive management—Strategies including pericardiocentesis/pericardial drainage should be considered in patients with symptomatic pericardial effusion/tamponade. VATS or balloon pericardiotomy may be warranted in those with significant risk of recurrence. Surgical pericardiectomy should be avoided due to the complexity and high risk associated with this procedure.

Management of Patients with Days to Weeks of Life Expectancy

- Medical management—Symptom management with opioids or other analgesics should be considered if traditional therapy is not tolerated or is insufficient for pain control in those with acute/recurrent pericarditis. Opioids may also have a role in the management of dyspnea in those with significant pericardial effusion/tamponade or in those with constrictive pericarditis.
- Invasive management—Drainage with catheter placement should be considered in highly symptomatic patients who have weeks of life expectancy. Further invasive management is discouraged as it may result in additional risk and discomfort with limited benefit.

Recommended Reading

1. Roy C, et al. Does this patient with a pericardial effusion have cardiac tamponade? *JAMA* 2007;297(16):1810–1818.

2. Maich B, et al. Guidelines on the diagnosis and management of pericardial diseases executive summary; The Task Force on the Diagnosis and Management of Pericardial Diseases of the European Society of Cardiology. *Eur Heart J* 2004;25(7):587.

3. Imazio M, et al. Management of pericardial effusion. *Eur Heart J* 2013;34(16):1186–1197.

Chapter 11

Arrhythmias

Masanori Mori

Classification

- Bradycardias—Sinus bradycardia, sick sinus syndrome (SSS)
- Atrioventricular (AV) block—First-degree, second-degree Mobitz I (Wenckebach), second-degree Mobitz II, third-degree (complete) AV block
- Supraventricular tachycardias (SVTs)
  - Atrial—Sinus tachycardia (ST), SA node reentrant tachycardia (SANRT), atrial tachycardia (AT), multifocal atrial tachycardia (MAT), atrial flutter (AFL), atrial fibrillation (AF)
  - AV junction—AV nodal reentrant tachycardia (AVNRT), atrioventricular reciprocating tachycardia (AVRT), nonparoxysmal junctional tachycardia (NPJT)
- Accessory pathways [Wolff–Parkinson–White (WPW)]—AVRT, AF with rapid conduction
- Wide-complex tachycardias (WCTs)—SVT conducted with aberrancy, ventricular tachycardia (VT)—monomorphic, polymorphic [e.g., torsades de pointes (TdP)]

Symptoms and Signs

- Palpitations, chest pain, dyspnea, lightheadedness, fatigue, heart failure, syncope

Investigations

- Blood tests to assess electrolytes (especially K, Mg), thyroid function, and anemia
- Electrocardiogram (ECG), 24-hour monitoring, CXR
- Echocardiogram to evaluate LV function and valve dysfunction
- Stress test or cardiac catheterization to rule out ischemia
- Electrophysiology study to assess inducibility

Management for Patients with Years of Life Expectancy

- SSS—Usually need both medications [β-blocker (BB), calcium channel blocker (CCB), digoxin] for tachycardia and permanent pacemaker (PPM) for bradycardia.
- AV block—No treatment required for first degree AV block and Wenckebach. PPM required for Mobitz II and complete AV block.
- Atrial fibrillation
  - Rate control can be achieved with CCB, β-blocker (BB), digoxin, and amiodarone.
  - Rhythm control has no clear survival benefit versus rate control.
  - Cardioversion may be considered for first AF episode or if symptomatic.
  - Anticoagulation, if indicated, should be used to prevent thromboemboli.
- SVTs
  - Consider treating underlying etiology for ST.
  - Cardioversion should be considered for unstable SVT patients.
  - BB, CCB, or amiodarone for AT and NPJT; BB, CCB, digoxin, and AAD for AF/AFL; and CCB or BB if tolerated for multifocal atrial tachycardia (MAT).
  - Vagal maneuvers, adenosine, CCB, or BB can be used for AVNRT or AVRT.
- WPW syndrome
  - AVRT—Vagal maneuvers, BB, CCB
  - AF/AFL with conduction down accessory pathway—Use procainamide, ibutilide, flecainide, or cardioversion. Avoid BB/CCB and digoxin/adenosine.
  - Long term: Radiofrequency ablation or antiarrhythmics (IA, IC)
- WCTs
  - Correct electrolytes (K, Mg) and use medications (BB and antiarrhythmics).
  - Consider implantable cardioverter-defibrillator (ICD) for secondary prevention after ventricular tachycardia/ventricular fibrillation (VT/VF) arrest and for primary prevention in high-risk patients. Radiofrequency ablation can be considered.

Relevance to the Cancer Palliative Care Setting

- Arrhythmias can cause significant symptom burden and interfere with activities of daily living (ADL). In patients with symptomatic arrhythmias and a reasonable life expectancy, appropriate cardiac work up and management may be warranted to maintain QOL.
- Cytotoxic agents can cause arrhythmias. Whereas paclitaxel can lead to bradycardia, ifosfamide, gemcitabine, melphalan, cisplatin, docetaxel, 5-fluorouracil, and etoposide and high-dose corticosteroids can induce AF. Targeted agents such as trastuzumab, pazopanib, and catamuxomab also have proarrhythmic effects.

- Antiarrhythmic agents such as amiodarone, flecainide, and quinidine are pro-arrhythmic as well, and they prolong the QT interval. When used in cancer patients on a multitude of other QT-prolonging medications (Table 11.1), the synergistic effect may be significant. Detection of high-risk patients with a history of cardiac diseases, correction of electrolyte abnormalities, and close ECG monitoring are important to decrease the risk of life-threatening arrhythmia such as TdP.

Management for Patients with Months of Life Expectancy

- Invasive procedures and interventions such as cardiac catheterization and PPM placement are not usually indicated at this stage.
- If symptomatic, noninvasive pharmacologic treatment may be appropriate.
- Anticoagulation for AF may need to be discontinued since risks of bleeding can overweigh its benefits.

Management for Patients with Weeks/Days of Life Expectancy

- Cardiac monitoring may not be necessary when the goal of care is patient comfort.
- Avoid frequent blood work if possible.
- Subcutaneous or intravenous morphine infusion may relieve dyspnea.
- Cardiopulmonary resuscitation in cancer patients with far advanced disease and cardiac arrest is futile and should not be recommended.

Table 11.1 Examples of Drugs Producing Prolonged QT Interval

Class	Drugs
Targeted agents	Dasatinib, nilotinib, pazopanib, sunitinib, vorinostat, vemurafenib
Antidepressants	Amitryptiline, clomipramine, desipramine, imipramine
Antibiotics	Clarithromycin, erythromycin, sparfloxacin, pentamidine
Antifungals	Ketoconazole, miconazole, itraconazole
Serotonin agonist/ antagonist	Cisapride, ketaserin, zimeldine
Antipsychotics	Chlorpromazine, droperidol, haloperidol
Antiemetics	Domperidone
Antiarrhythmics	IA: procainamide, quinidine, amaline, disopyramide
	IB: flecaine, propafenvone
	III: amiodarone, sotalol, dofetilide, ibutilide
Vasodilators	Bepridil, perhexiline
Other	Methadone

Recommended Reading

1. Sabatine MS. *Pocket Medicine (4th ed.)*. Lippincott Williams & Wilkins, Baltimore, MD, 2011.

2. Svoboda M, et al. Cardiac toxicity of targeted therapies used in the treatment for solid tumors: a review. *Cardiovasc Toxicol* 2012;12(3):191–207.

3. Brana I, et al. Cardiotoxicity. *Ann Oncol* 2010;21(Suppl 7):vii173–vii179.

4. Chen CL, Parameswaran R. Managing the risks and cardiac therapy in cancer patients. *Semin Oncol* 2013;40(2):210–217.

Chapter 12

Arterial Hypertension

Caroline Ha

Classification

- Prehypertension—Systolic 120–139 mmHg or diastolic 80–89 mmHg
- Primary hypertension
  - Stage 1 hypertension—Systolic 140–159 mmHg or diastolic 90–99 mmHg
  - Stage 2 hypertension—Systolic ≥160 mmHg or diastolic ≥100 mmHg
  - Hypertensive urgency—Systolic ≥180 mmHg or diastolic ≥120 mmHg. It is often symptomatic but without evidence of progressive target organ dysfunction.
  - Hypertensive emergency—Systolic ≥180 mmHg or diastolic ≥120 mmHg. There is evidence of progressive target organ dysfunction.
- Secondary hypertension—Chronic kidney disease, aortic coarctation, Cushing's syndrome, chronic steroid therapy, medication side effect, pheochromocytoma, primary aldosteronism, renovascular hypertension, sleep apnea, and hyperthyroidism

Symptoms and Signs

- Symptoms—Hypertension is usually asymptomatic. However, a hypertensive urgency or emergency may be associated with headache, dyspnea, epistaxis, severe anxiety, chest pain, nausea and vomiting, paresthesias, dizziness, and altered mental status.
- Signs—Arrhythmias and focal neurological signs may occur in hypertensive emergency.

Investigations

- Routine tests recommended before initiating therapy include a 12-lead electrocardiogram, serum potassium, estimated glomerular filtration rate (or creatinine), blood glucose, hematocrit, serum calcium, urinalysis, and a fasting lipoprotein profile. Urinary albumin excretion or albumin/creatinine ratio should be measured in patients with diabetes or renal disease.
- Tests for secondary causes are optional and can be considered if:
  - Hypertension proves resistant to treatment.
  - Clinical examination or routine tests suggest a secondary cause.

Relevance to the Cancer Palliative Care Setting

- Hypertension has a high prevalence in the general population, affecting over half of people aged 60–69 years and three of four people aged 70 and over. Many cancer patients have comorbid hypertension.
- Cachexia resulting from cancer can cause significant reductions in weight, which can decrease blood pressure. Cancer can also contribute to autonomic dysfunction. Thus, antihypertensive doses may need to be reduced to prevent hypotension, dizziness, fainting, and falls.
- Targeted agents affecting the vascular endothelial growth factor receptor (VEGFR) pathway such as bevacizumab, sorafenib, sunitinib, axitinib, and pazopanib are associated with an increased risk of hypertension.

Management for Patients with Years of Life Expectancy

- Hypertension—Reduction of blood pressure to <140/90 mmHg (or <130/80 mmHg for patients with comorbid diabetes or renal disease) has been found to reduce mortality from ischemic heart disease and stroke. Antihypertensive medications should be used if lifestyle modifications (Table 12.1) alone are insufficient to achieve the blood pressure goal. Thiazide diuretics have robust data showing reduction in cardiovascular risk and are the

Table 12.1 Lifestyle Modifications to Prevent and Manage Hypertension*

Modification	Recommendation	Approximate Systolic Blood Pressure Reduction (Range)
Weight reduction	Maintain normal body weight (body mass index 18.5–24.9 kg/m²).	5–20 mmHg/10kg
Adopt Dietary Approaches to Stop Hypertension (DASH) eating plan	Consume a diet rich in fruits, vegetables, and low-fat dairy products with a reduced content of saturated and total fat.	8–14 mmHg
Dietary sodium reduction	Reduce dietary sodium intake to no more than 100 mmol per day (2.4 g sodium or 6 g sodium chloride).	2–8 mmHg
Physical activity	Engage in regular aerobic physical activity such as brisk walking (at least 30 min per day, most days of the week).	4–9 mmHg
Moderation of alcohol consumption	Limit consumption to no more than two drinks (e.g., 24 oz beer, 10 oz wine, or 3 oz 80-proof whiskey) per day in most men, and to no more than one drink per day in women and lighter weight persons.	2–4 mmHg

*For overall cardiovascular risk reduction, stop smoking.
Source: National Heart, Lung, and Blood Institute; National Institutes of Health; U.S. Department of Health and Human Services.

preferred initial agents for most patients. Indications for initiating treatment with other agents are presented in Table 12.2 and the doses are listed in Table 12.3.

- Hypertensive emergency—Admission to an intensive care unit for continuous blood pressure monitoring and parenteral antihypertensive medication treatment is indicated. Rapid falls in blood pressure can precipitate renal, cerebral, or coronary ischemia; therefore, treatment should proceed as follows:
  - First hour: Reduce mean arterial blood pressure (MAP) by no more than 25%.
  - Hours 2–6: Reduce blood pressure to 160/100–110 mmHg if the patient is stable.

Management for Patients with Months of Life Expectancy

- In patients with hypertension other than urgency or emergency, there is inadequate evidence that blood pressure reduction is beneficial. Therefore, the focus of antihypertensive treatment should shift to quality of life.

Table 12.2 Antihypertensive Usage in Comorbidities and Selected Adverse Effects

Medication Class	Strong Indications for Use in	Selected Adverse Effects
Diuretic	Heart failure High coronary artery disease risk Diabetes mellitus Recurrent stroke prevention	Hypokalemia Hyponatremia Urinary frequency Gout
β-Blocker	Heart failure Post-myocardial infarction High coronary artery disease risk Diabetes mellitus	Fatigue Depression Heart block
Angiotensin-converting enzyme (ACE) inhibitor	Heart failure Post-myocardial infarction High coronary artery disease risk Diabetes mellitus Chronic kidney disease Recurrent stroke prevention	Renal impairment Angioedema Cough Hyperkalemia
Angiotensin receptor blocker	Heart failure Diabetes mellitus Chronic kidney disease	Similar to ACE-I, but lower incidence of cough
Calcium channel blocker	High coronary artery disease risk Diabetes mellitus	Ankle edema Heart block Headache Flushing
Aldosterone antagonist	Heart failure Post-myocardial infarction	Hyperkalemia Urinary frequency Gynecomastia Impotence

Source: National Heart, Lung, and Blood Institute; National Institutes of Health; U.S. Department of Health and Human Services.

Table 12.3 Pharmacologic Therapy for Hypertension

Class	Common Medications and Doses
Diuretic	Hydrochlorothiazide 12.5 or 25 mg PO daily
	Chlorthalidone 12.5 or 25 mg PO daily
	Furosemide 20 mg PO daily
β-Blocker	Metoprolol 25 or 50 mg PO BID
	Metoprolol extended release 25 or 50 mg PO daily
	Carvedilol 3.125, 6.25, 12.5, or 25 mg PO Q12h
Angiotensin-converting enzyme inhibitor	Enalapril 5, 10, or 20 mg PO daily
	Lisinopril 10 or 20 mg PO daily
	Ramipril 2.5, 5, or 10 mg PO daily
Angiotensin receptor blocker	Irbesartan 150 or 300 mg PO daily
	Losartan 25 or 50 mg PO daily
	Olmesartan 20 or 40 mg PO daily
	Valsartan 80 or 160 mg PO daily
Calcium channel blocker	Diltiazem extended release 120, 180, or 240 mg PO daily
	Amlodipine 2.5, 5, or 10 mg PO daily
	Nifedipine long-acting 30 or 60 mg PO daily
	Nicardipine sustained release 30 or 60 mg PO BID

- Limit further diagnostic and laboratory studies for hypertension whenever possible.
- Consider liberalizing the patient's diet.
- Discontinue or reduce antihypertensive medications if the patient experiences bothersome side effects, has orthostatic hypotension, or desires to take fewer medications.
- Hypertensive urgency and emergency—Management is similar to that of patients with years of life expectancy, unless the patient does not desire hospitalization.

Management for Patients with Weeks/Days of Life Expectancy

- Patients may be unable to take oral medications. In addition, hypotension is common in dying patients. Blood pressure treatment should be discontinued unless the patient has symptoms from severely elevated blood pressure.

Recommended Reading

1. Chobanian AV, Bakris GL, Black HR, et al. Seventh report of the Joint National Committee on prevention, detection, evaluation, and treatment of high blood pressure. *Hypertension* 2003;42(6):1206–1252.

2. Kotchen TA. Hypertensive vascular disease. In Longo DL, Fauci AS, Kasper DL, et al. (eds.), *Harrison's Principles of Internal Medicine* (18th ed.). McGraw-Hill Professional, New York, 2011: 2042–2059.

Chapter 13

Dyslipidemia

Holly M. Holmes

Classification

- Based on type of lipid abnormality
  - Hyperlipidemia: Elevated low-density lipoprotein (LDL)
  - Hypertriglyceridemia: Elevated triglycerides
  - Low high-density lipoprotein (HDL)
  - Mixed: High LDL and triglycerides
- Genetic classifications
  - Single gene defects, for example, familial hypercholesterolemia, with a defect on chromosome 19 and mutations in the LDL receptor gene
  - Polygenic defects
  - Genetic defects plus environmental factors, and secondary to other comorbid conditions (e.g., diabetes mellitus)

Epidemiology

- Dyslipidemia is a significant risk factor for cardiovascular disease (CVD), the leading cause of death in the Unites States.
- In the United States 53.4% of adults have high cholesterol and 32% have high LDL.

Symptoms and Signs

- Symptoms—Generally a chronic, asymptomatic condition, but dyslipidemia is associated with vascular disease, which may be symptomatic.
- Signs—Few signs, but when markedly elevated, there may be xanthomas (cholesterol deposits on tendons and in soft tissues) and xanthelasmas (cholesterol deposits on the eyelids).

Investigations

- For initial screening, the US Preventive Services Task Force 2008 guidelines strongly recommend screening all men 35 years and older and women 45 years and older who are at increased risk of CVD.
  - Initial screening consists of a total cholesterol level and, if possible, with a measurement of HDL.

- Increased risk for CVD is defined by the following:
  - History of diabetes mellitus
  - Prior coronary heart disease or noncoronary atherosclerotic disease
  - Family history of CVD in men younger than 50 years or women younger than 60 years
  - Tobacco use
  - Hypertension
  - Obesity
- Abnormal screening tests should be followed by full lipid panel measurement (total cholesterol, LDL, HDL, and triglycerides) to further determine risk and therapeutic strategy (see Table 13.1).

Relevance to the Cancer Palliative Care Setting

- Treatment of dyslipidemia may contribute to nonspecific symptoms that may diminish quality of life.
  - Palliative care patients may be at higher risk of developing myalgia due to lipid-lowering therapy.
- Drug interactions in dyslipidemia are common but of uncertain clinical significance.
  - Many medications inhibit the metabolism of statins, thus increasing statin levels and increasing the risk for myalgia and myopathy.
  - Combination lipid therapy (e.g., statins plus ezetimibe) increases the risk of myalgia.

Management of Patients with Years of Life Expectancy

- Treatment of dyslipidemia and the goals of therapy are based on the estimation of cardiac risk (Table 13.1), with 10-year cardiac risk typically calculated using risk estimators such as the Framingham score.

Table 13.1 Current Guidelines Regarding the Management of Dyslipidemia*

Category Based on Risk Factors	LDL Goal	LDL Level to Initiate Drug Therapy
High risk: CVD or equivalent or 10-year risk of >20%	<100 mg/dL <70 mg/dL if very high risk	LDL ≥100 mg/dL
Moderately high risk: ≥ 2 risk factors or 10-year risk of 10–20%	<130 mg/dL	LDL ≥130 mg/dL
Moderate risk: ≥ 2 risk factors or 10-year risk of <10%	<130 mg/dL	LDL ≥160 mg/dL
Low risk: 1 or no risk factors	<160 mg/dL	LDL ≥190 mg/dL
* Based on the National Cholesterol Education Program, Adult Treatment Panel III Guidelines.		

- Lifestyle modification (diet and exercise) is initiated as part of treatment and may be the only initial treatment in individuals with dyslipidemia who do not meet the LDL threshold to initiate drug therapy.
- Primary prevention involves the treatment of dyslipidemia before any evidence of CVD. Treatment with statins (HMG CoA reductase inhibitors) is recommended (Table 13.2), but other nonstatin medications may be used (such as ezetimibe, bile-acid binders, fibric acid derivatives, and omega fatty acids). The evidence of benefit in primary prevention is strongest for statin medications but is not consistent across subpopulations, including older persons and women.
- For secondary prevention, statins are indicated in patients with a history of CVD, with a number needed to treat (NNT) of 50 for the reduction of all-cause mortality at 5 years in people with a history of CVD.
- Management of other cardiac risk factors should also be used in conjunction with medication, including smoking cessation, weight loss, exercise, and dietary modification.

Management for Patients with Months of Life Expectancy

- Management is somewhat controversial. Continuation or initiation of lipid-lowering therapy depends greatly on cardiac risk and individual patient and family preference.

Table 13.2 Pharmacologic Therapy for Dyslipidemia

Class	Common Medications and Doses
Statins (HMG CoA reductase inhibitors)	Atorvastatin 10 to 80 mg once daily, may be given at any time of day
	Simvastatin 5 to 40 mg once daily in the evening, use 80 mg daily only in patients tolerating this dose for at least 1 year, dose adjustment in the presence of drug interactions
	Rosuvastatin 5 to 40 mg once daily, may be given at any time of day
	Pravastatin 10 to 80 mg once daily in the evening
	Fluvastatin 10 to 80 mg once daily in the evening
	Lovastatin 10 to 80 mg once daily in the evening, dose adjustment in the presence of drug interactions
Fibric acid derivatives	Gemfibrozil 600 mg twice daily
	Fenofibrate 40 to 200 mg daily (depending on formulation)
	Fenofibric acid 35 to 135 mg daily
Niacin	Niacin regular release 250 mg to 6 g daily
	Niacin sustained release 1 to 2 g daily
	Niacin extended release 500 mg at bedtime, up to 2 g daily
Ezetimibe	Ezetimibe 10 mg daily
Bile acid sequestrants	Cholestyramine 4 g once to twice daily, maximum 24 g daily
	Colesevelam 1.875 g twice daily, maximum 4.375 g daily
	Colestipol granules 5 g once to twice daily, up to 30 g daily
	Colestipol tablets 2 g once to twice daily, up to 16 g daily

- Patients with a recent cardiovascular or cerebrovascular event are at higher baseline risk of a recurrent event and derive a higher benefit from statin. For those with a recent cardiac or cerebrovascular event or acute coronary syndrome, use of a statin may be warranted despite diminishing remaining life expectancy.
- In individuals receiving statins for primary prevention, statin discontinuation should be considered in light of patients' preferences for continuing therapy. Patients may want to continue therapy as part of a health maintenance strategy or to avoid a feeling of abandonment.
- Relaxed lipid targets may be more reasonable, particularly in patients with low to moderate risk of CVD.
- In older persons, lower lipid levels are associated with increased mortality.

Management for Patients with Weeks/Days of Life Expectancy

- The benefit of prevention, particularly primary prevention, is not likely to be achieved for this patient population.
- The benefits and risks of treatment of dyslipidemia in hospice settings are unknown.
  - The effect of statins on common symptoms, such as angina, is unknown.
  - It is possible that continued treatment of high-risk individuals could reduce symptoms of CVD.
- Although the harms of continuing medication may be uncertain, stopping may be reasonable, particularly if taking the medication is burdensome or costly.
- Avoid checking lipid levels in these patients.

Recommended Reading

1. Last AR, Ference JD, Falleroni, J. Pharmacologic treatment of hyperlipidemia. *Am Fam Physician* 2011;84:551–558.
2. Vollrath AM, Sinclair C, Hallenbeck C. Discontinuing cardiovascular medications at the end of life: lipid-lowering agents. *J Palliat Med* 2005;8:876–881.

Section IV

Nephrology and Metabolic Abnormalities

Chapter 14

Chronic Kidney Disease and Acute Kidney Injury

Jane O. Schell and Robert M. Arnold

Classification and Causes

- Acute kidney injury (AKI)
  - AKI is defined as an abrupt loss of kidney function with subsequent rise in serum creatinine and/or a decrease in urine output.
  - Causes of AKI include:
    - Prerenal—Volume depletion, hypotensive insults (sepsis, infection)
    - Intrinsic—Direct involvement of the tumor or indirect damage from ischemic insults, drug toxicity, or tumor-related processes
    - Postobstructive—External or internal compression of the urinary outflow tract
- Chronic kidney disease (CKD) is a common finding in cancer patients due to advanced age and underlying comorbidities (e.g., hypertension, ischemic injury). Early recognition of CKD can enhance the awareness and management of at-risk patients for renal injury.

Symptoms and Signs

- Symptoms in AKI and CKD are common and independent of cancer diagnosis.
  - AKI presents typically with weakness, light-headedness, complaints of thirst and dehydration, and confusion.
  - CKD symptoms include pruritus, fatigue, insomnia, depression, and pain.
  - Pain is reported in >50% of dialysis patients with the predominant case musculoskeletal.
  - Other causes include pain related to underlying comorbidities, such as diabetes, dialysis-related symptoms (interdialytic hypotension, cramping), ischemic pain related to dialysis access, bone mineral abnormalities, and pain related to underlying cancer.
- Signs include hypotension, signs of hypervolemia or hypovolemia, asterixis, altered mental status, decreased urine output, and electrolyte abnormalities.

Investigations

- Serum creatinine is typically used as a marker of renal injury, although it has significant limitations. Renal function should be estimated by calculation [Cockcroft–Gault or abbreviated Modification of Diet in Renal Disease (MDRD) equations] or measured by 24-hour urine collection. These estimations take into account age, sex, race, and body size.
- RIFLE criteria (Risk, Injury, Failure, Loss, End-Stage Renal Disease) estimate levels of kidney injury based on elevation in serum creatinine and changes in urine output (Table 14.1).

Relevance to the Cancer Palliative Care Setting

- Patients with cancer are three times more likely to experience AKI compared to those without cancer. The rate of AKI in hospitalized patients ranges from 12% at admission to 55% throughout the hospitalization.
- Patients with cancer and kidney disease experience considerable burdens and are at increased risk for poor outcomes.
- Outcomes in critically ill cancer patients with AKI are poor. The presence of AKI and the degree of injury are independent risk factors for mortality. Outcomes following dialysis initiation are impacted by health factors other than cancer diagnosis such as age, performance status, and health condition.
- Palliative care services can assist with symptom management and dialysis decision making. Hospice services can assist with the management of patients when the patient's goals shift from a focus on curative treatments toward one of comfort and quality of life.

Management of Patients with Years of Life Expectancy

- Management of cancer patients with years of life expectancy is similar to those with AKI or CKD without cancer. Care typically involves minimizing

Table 14.1 Rifle Criteria: Classification of Acute Kidney Injury and Outcomes
Risk—1.5-fold increase in the serum creatinine or glomerular filtration rate (GFR) decrease by 25% or urine output <0.5 mL/kg/h for 6 h
Injury—2-fold increase in the serum creatinine or GFR decrease by 50% or urine output <0.5 mL/kg/h for 12 h
Failure—3-fold increase in the serum creatinine or GFR decrease by 75% or urine output of <0.3 mL/kg/h for 24 h, or anuria for 12 h
Loss—Complete loss of kidney function (e.g., need for renal replacement therapy) for more than 4 weeks
End stage renal disease—Complete loss of kidney function (e.g., need for renal replacement therapy) for more than 3 months

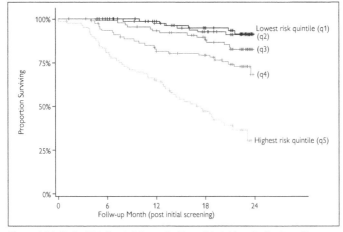

Figure 14.1 Kaplan Meir Survival Curves by Hemodialysis Mortality Predictor Score.

further kidney injury, management of fluid and electrolytes, and addressing anemia and bone mineral disease.

- Dialysis decision making is common in these patients whether following AKI or progressive CKD. Prognosis typically depends on the type and extent of cancer.

- Other important prognostic factors include nutritional status (serum albumin), functional status, severity of comorbidities (vascular disease, dementia), and elderly age.

- A hemodialysis (HD) mortality predictor uses a clinician's prediction plus five variables to predict 6-month and 12-month survival in hemodialysis patients (Figure 14.1). This integrated prognostic model is available on touchcalc: http://touchcalc.com/calculators/sq.

Management of Patients with Months of Life Expectancy

- Management of patients with months of life expectancy involves weighing the risks and benefits of dialysis and the potential impact on survival and quality of life.

- Dialysis decision making in these patients is best accomplished by eliciting the patient's goals and values. By understanding these *big picture* goals, the clinician can better determine whether dialysis is likely to achieve these goals and whether it is consistent with these goals.

  - Gaining an understanding of the patients goals and values—This understanding is best elicited though open-ended questions exploring the patient's understanding of disease, hopes for the future, and concerns that may influence decision making (Box 14.1).

Box 14.1 Gaining an Understanding of the Patient's Goals and Values

Invitation to assess the readiness to have a conversation:
"Can we talk about how things have been going?"

Using open-ended "big picture" questions to assess care goals and preferences:
"What is life like outside the hospital?"
"What is most important to you now?"
"What are you hoping for?"
Outline barriers to decision making:
"As you think about the future what worries you the most?"

Propose a plan that meets the patient's goals:
"Now that I understand your situation, can I make a recommendation?"

- Conversations about the future and overall prognosis often arouse feelings of uncertainty and emotion. The clinician's ability to recognize and respond to patient's affect can impact a patient's ability to process and meaningfully participate in discussions (Box 14.2).
- After consideration of the facts and of the patient's *big picture* goals, the clinical can provide a recommendation regarding dialysis that considers the balance of potential benefits and burdens of dialysis.
- When uncertainty exists, this decision may be to propose a time-limited trial of dialysis with opportunities to reassess clinical milestones and whether dialysis is assisting with these goals.

Box 14.2 Empathic Responses to Affective Concerns

Responding to emotional concerns (verbal empathy): N-U-R-S-E

Name the emotion: "You seem worried."
Understand: "I see why you are concerned about this."
Respect: "You have shown a lot of strength."
Support: "We will get through this together."
Explore: "Tell me more."

Responding to uncertainty:

Name the uncertainty
Respond to emotional response
Offer support: "What can we do for you given that we don't know for sure how things will go?"
Reaffirm your commitment: "I'll stick with you throughout this."

Management of Patients with Days/Weeks of Life Expectancy

- As patients experience clinical decline, they may experience more burdens of kidney disease and dialysis (if initiated). These burdens include weakness, lethargy, and difficulty tolerating treatments, including chemotherapy or dialysis.
- At end of life, symptoms tend to be similar to other terminal disease states with the greatest symptoms being pain, pruritus, shortness of breath, and agitation.
- Morphine should be avoided in the presence of kidney disease. Its principal metabolite morphine-3-glucuronide has neuroexcitatory effects that may contribute to myoclonus and opioid-induced neurotoxicity.
- Death occurs approximately 3–14 days after dialysis is withdrawn.

Recommended Reading

1. Aapro M, Launay-Vacher V. Importance of monitoring renal function in patients with cancer. *Cancer Treat Rev* 2012;38(3):235–240.
2. Cohen LM, Ruthazer R, Moss AH, Germain MJ. Predicting six-month mortality for patients who are on maintenance hemodialysis. *Clin J Am Soc Nephrol: CJASN* 2010;5(1):72–79.

Chapter 15

Urinary Incontinence

Akhila Reddy

Classification

- Transient Incontinence: Involuntary leakage of urine that ceases spontaneously after the underlying cause is resolved. The causes include delirium, urinary tract infections, atrophic vaginitis, medications such as diuretics, excessive urine output from conditions such as congestive heart failure and hyperglycemia, fecal impaction, pregnancy, and psychological disorders.
- Chronic Urinary Incontinence. See Table 15.1.

Assessments

- A thorough patient history to assess voiding symptoms, medical, urologic, and gynecologic conditions including previous surgeries.
- Rule out any reversible causes that could lead to transient incontinence.
- Physical examination should include a pelvic or prostate and rectal examination.
- Cough stress test may help to confirm the diagnosis of stress incontinence.
- Measure postvoid residual urine if overflow incontinence is suspected.
- Voiding diary.

Investigations

- Urine analysis and serum creatinine
- Prostate-specific antigen testing may be considered in men if symptoms or physical examination indicate a prostate etiology.

Relevance to the Cancer Palliative Care Setting

- Radical prostatectomy is the most common cause of stress incontinence in men.
- Prior pelvic surgeries or radiation for gynecologic or genitourinary cancers may give rise to stress, urge, and mixed incontinence.
- Tumor involvement of sacral nerves may result in symptoms of urge incontinence.

- Functional incontinence is often seen in patients with advanced cancer who have decreased mobility.
- Anticholinergics can precipitate delirium in the cancer palliative setting.
- Be mindful of all the side effects and drug interactions of the pharmacologic treatments of incontinence in patients with advanced cancer.

Table 15.1 Types of Chronic Urinary Incontinence			
Type	**Pathophysiology**	**Associated Factors**	**Signs and Symptoms**
Stress	Weakness of urethral sphincter/pelvic floor, neurogenic weakness of urethral sphincter	Damage to pelvic muscles, nerves, and fascia (e.g., radical prostatectomy or transurethral resection of the prostate), neurogenic causes (e.g., myelomeningocele); most common in younger women.	Leakage of urine with physical exertion or increase in intraabdominal pressure such as coughing or sneezing
Urge	Detrusor overactivity as a result of intrinsic bladder causes or loss of neurologic control of bladder contractions	Associated with stroke, multiple sclerosis, and other neurologic disorders; may also be associated with overflow and stress incontinence; most common in older adults	Leakage of urine associated with a sudden strong urge to void; leakage of urine usually happens on the way to the toilet
Mixed	Incontinence overlapping detrusor overactivity along with impaired urethral sphincter function	Is the cause in up to 30% of the patients with chronic urinary incontinence	Involuntary leakage associated with sudden urgency and also with physical exertion and increase in intraabdominal pressure
Overflow	Overdistension of bladder and related leakage of urine caused by impaired detrusor contractility, bladder outlet obstruction, or neurologic disorders	Associated with neurogenic bladder, idiopathic detrusor failure, urethral stricture, prostate diseases, post-pelvic surgery or radiation	Dribbling or continuous leakage of urine, incomplete bladder emptying, weak urinary stream, hesitancy, frequency, and nocturia
Functional	Functional, cognitive, or psychological impairment causing a barrier to toileting and causing leakage of urine	Associated with conditions such as arthritis, advanced cancer, dementia, cerebral vascular accident, gait disturbance, or psychiatric conditions	Nongenitourinary factors such as cognitive impairment and immobility that interfere with the patient's ability to void independently

Management for Patients with Years of Life Expectancy

- Treat the underlying reversible causes if transient incontinence is suspected.
- Lifestyle changes: Weight loss, smoking cessation, limiting excessive fluid intake, and avoidance of caffeinated and alcoholic beverages.
- Behavioral therapy: Bladder training, pelvic muscle exercises, and biofeedback can be effective in the management of stress, urge, and mixed incontinence.
- Pharmacologic management: Although not approved for this purpose in the United States, duloxetine, a serotonin and norepinephrine reuptake inhibitor, may be effective in stress incontinence, and local topical estrogen in the form of vaginal creams, rings, or dissolvable tablets may improve symptoms of incontinence in women with vaginal atrophy. See Table 15.2 for more details.

Table 15.2 Pharmacologic Therapy for Urinary Incontinence

Drug	Common Medications and Doses	Side Effects	Uses
Anticholinergic drugs	Oxybutynin (5 mg immediate release BID–TID or 5–15 mg extended release once daily) Tolterodine (1–2 mg immediate release BID or 2–4 mg extended release once daily) Fesoterodine (4–8 mg extended release once daily) Trospium (20 mg immediate release BID or 60 mg extended release once daily) Darifenacin (7.5–15 mg extended release once daily) Solifenacin (5–10 mg once daily)	Dry mouth, blurred vision, tachycardia, drowsiness, cognitive impairment, and constipation	Urge and mixed incontinence
β-Adrenergic agonists	Mirabegron (25–50 mg extended release once daily)	Nausea, diarrhea, fatigue, headache, tachycardia, hypertension, and nasopharyngitis	Urge incontinence
α-Adrenergic antagonists	Tamsulosin (0.4–0.8 mg once daily at bedtime) Alfuzosin (10 mg once daily at bedtime) Terazosin (1–10 mg once daily at bedtime) Doxazosin (1–8 mg once daily at bedtime)	Orthostatic hypotension and dizziness	Urge incontinence in men associated with poor emptying of the bladder
Botulinum toxin A	(Injected into the detrusor muscle every 3–6 months)	Posttreatment urinary retention	Urge incontinence refractory to behavior therapy and anticholinergic drugs

- Surgery: Neuromodulation with sacral nerve stimulator can be helpful in intractable urge incontinence. Sling procedures such as suburethral, pubo-vaginal, and mid urethral slings along with retropubic colposuspension or urethropexy and periurethral injections of bulking agents are all potential options for stress incontinence in women.

Management for Patients with Months of Life Expectancy

- Lifestyle changes, behavior therapy, and pharmacologic treatments are generally indicated.
- Surgical options may pose more risk than benefit and are generally not indicated.
- Mechanical devices such as pessary and urethral plugs may be used to manage stress incontinence.

Management for Patients with Weeks/Days of Life Expectancy

- Pharmacologic treatment may be attempted if oral or transdermal routes are an option.
- Pads, protective garments, and indwelling urethral catheter may be considered for these patients.

Recommended Reading

1. Gormley EA, Lightner DJ, Burgio KL, et al. Diagnosis and treatment of over-active bladder (non-neurogenic) in adults: AUA/SUFU guideline. *J Urol* 2012;188(6 Suppl):2455–2463.
2. Rai BP, et al. Anticholinergic drugs versus non-drug active therapies for non-neurogenic overactive bladder syndrome in adults. *Cochrane Database Syst Rev* 2012;12:CD003193.

Chapter 16

Urinary Retention

Akhila Reddy

Classification

- Acute urinary retention—Sudden inability to void despite having a full bladder.
- Chronic urinary retention—Urinary retention associated with increased volume of residual urine.

Causes

- Obstruction—Benign prostatic hyperplasia, prostate cancer, cystocele, rectocele, pelvic mass, gynecologic malignancy, bladder calculi, bladder neoplasm, fecal impaction, and retroperitoneal mass
- Inflammatory—Prostatitis, prostatic abscess, vulvovaginitis, cystitis, urethritis, and vaginal lichen sclerosis
- Pharmacological—Opioid analgesics, α-adrenergic agents, β-adrenergic agents, tricyclic antidepressants, anticholinergics, neuroleptics, antihistamines, muscle relaxants, calcium channel blockers
- Neurological—Disk herniation, spinal cord compression from tumors, tumors in the brain, multiple sclerosis, normal pressure hydrocephalus, radical pelvic surgery, cerebrovascular disease, and hematoma or abscesses of the spinal cord and diabetic neuropathy
- Other causes—Postoperative, trauma, and pregnancy-associated urinary retention

Symptoms and Signs

- Symptoms—May have obstructive symptoms such as urinary frequency, urgency, nocturia, straining to void, hesitancy, sensation of incomplete voiding, pelvic pressure, lower abdominal pain, hematuria and constipation. Fever, dysuria, back pain, perineal pain, urinary frequency, and urethral discharge may also be detected if an inflammatory etiology is present. History of overflow incontinence with neurologic causes.

Investigations

- Thorough history to include current symptoms, past medical and surgical history, history of radiation, medication use, and review of systems.
- Complete physical examination with focus on abdominal, pelvic, rectal, and neurologic examination.
- Measure postvoid residual urine in suspected chronic urinary retention.
- Urine analysis, serum blood urea nitrogen, creatinine, electrolytes, glucose, prostate-specific antigen.
- Pelvic ultrasound, computed tomograghy, and magnetic resonance imaging of the abdomen, pelvis, brain, and spinal cord are indicated if a neoplasm or neurologic etiology is suspected.

Management for Patients with Years of Life Expectancy

- Immediate decompression of the bladder through catheterization in acute urinary retention; suprapubic catheterization in cases in which urethral catheterization is contraindicated (e.g., recent radical prostatectomy or urethral reconstruction).
- Hospitalization is recommended for conditions such as spinal cord compression, malignancy-related obstruction, or urosepsis.
- Treatment with α-adrenergic blockers (tamsulosin, alfuzosin, and doxazosin) may lead to a greater chance of a successful voiding trial without a catheter in a patient with benign prostatic hypertrophy, which is the most common cause of urinary retention (Table 16.1).
- Prevention of acute urinary retention can be accomplished by long-term treatment with dutasteride or finasteride in benign prostatic hypertrophy.
- Surgical options are available depending upon the etiology for urinary retention such as transurethral resection of the prostate in benign prostatic hypertrophy.

Table 16.1 Pharmacologic Therapy for Urinary Retention	
Class	**Common Medications and Doses**
α-Adrenergic blockers*	Terazosin starting dose of 1 mg/day, can titrate slowly over 7 weeks to 10 mg/day
	Doxazosin starting dose of 1 mg/day, can titrate slowly over 4–8 weeks to 8 mg/day
	Alfuzosin 10 mg/day
	Tamsulosin starting dose of 0.4 mg/day, can titrate to 0.8 mg/day in 2–4 weeks
5 α-Reductase inhibitors	Finasteride 5 mg once daily
	Dutasteride 0.5 mg once daily
* Titrate doses to reduce orthostatic hypotension-related side effects. Medication is to be administered once daily at bedtime.	

- Clean intermittent catheterization is preferred over indwelling catheters to avoid complications such as upper urinary tract infections, sepsis, and renal failure in chronic urinary retention.
- Definitive management of urinary retention depends upon treating the underlying cause with both medical and/or surgical options.

Relevance to the Cancer Palliative Care Setting

- Urinary retention (acute and chronic) may occur as a result of genitourinary and gynecologic cancers, pelvic surgeries, prostate surgeries, radiation to the pelvic area, cancer in the brain or spine, and medications such as opioids that are commonly used in the advanced cancer population.
- Management of urinary retention secondary to opioids may involve the administration of naloxone or naltrexone in severe cases. The role for opioid rotation or opioid dose reduction is unclear.

Management for Patients with Months of Life Expectancy

- Management is similar to patients with years of life expectancy.
- Hospitalization is indicated in urinary retention associated with malignancy.
- Surgical options may pose more risk than benefit and are generally not indicated.

Management for Patients with Weeks/Days of Life Expectancy

- Oral medications may not be possible due to possible dysphagia at end of life.
- An indwelling urethral catheter is preferred over intermittent catheterization.

Recommended Reading

1. Selius BA, Subedi R. Urinary retention in adults: diagnosis and initial management. *Am Fam Physician* 2008;77(5):643–650.
2. Negro CL, Muir GH. Chronic urinary retention in men: how we define it, and how does it affect treatment outcome. *BJU Int* 2012;110(11):1590–1594.

Chapter 17

Hematuria

Meiko Kuriya

Definition

- Hematuria may be macroscopic (grossly visible) or microscopic (detectable only on urine examination).

Etiologies

- Inflammation—Cystitis (urinary tract infection, radiation cystitis, and cyclophosphamide-induced cystitis), urethritis, prostitis, or pyelonephritis
- Glomerulonephritis
- Trauma—Foley, surgery
- Nephrolithiasis
- Vascular—Renal infarction or renal vein thrombosis
- Malignancy of the kidney or urinary tract

Investigations

- Complete blood count (CBC) with differential, electrolytes, blood urea nitrogen/creatinine (BUN/Cr), urinalysis, urine culture and sensitivity (C&S), international normalized ratio/partial thromboplastin time (INR/PTT)
- Image study; kidney, ureter, and bladder (KUB) if nephrolithiasis is suspected, ultrasonography if obstruction suspected, computed tomography (CT) or cystoscopy if malignancy is suspected or if follow-up of known malignancy is necessary
- Urine cytology or biopsy if clinically indicated

Relevance to the Cancer Palliative Care Setting

- Hematuria may occur as a result of cancer treatments such as radiation therapy or administration of cyclophosphamide.
- Cancer patients may be on anticoagulants, which may predispose them to bleeding.

Management for Patients with Years of Life Expectancy

• Transurethral resection or palliative cystectomy may be indicated in severe cases of gross hematuria related to bladder tumor.
• If hematuria is microscopic, urinalysis should be rechecked in 6 weeks. Patients with persistent hematuria should undergo a thorough work-up to determine the etiology and treat accordingly.

Management for Patients with Months of Life Expectancy

• Management is similar to patients with years of life expectancy.
• If hematuria is persistent and bladder tumor is unresectable, urinary diversion or embolization may be considered.
• Patients with urinary tract infection should be treated with antibiotics.
• For persistent hematuria, follow Hb as well as clinical signs of anemia. Transfuse if clinically indicated.

Management for Patients with Weeks/Days of Life Expectancy

• Invasive procedures such as biopsy may be avoided depending on the patients' condition and remaining life expectancy, especially if the biopsy result will not change the overall management plan.
• If a risk of blood clot causing urinary obstruction is present, place a urethral catheter and continuously irrigate the bladder with normal saline.
• Aminocaproic acid, intravesical formalin, alum or prostaglandin irrigation, hydrostatic pressure, and radiotherapy represent potential treatment options for intractable hematuria from bladder cancer, although well-designed studies are lacking.
• Avoid tranexamic acid in patients with bladder hemorrhage because it may predispose to clot formation in the urinary tract.

Recommended Reading

1. Schultz M, van der Lelie H. Microscopic haematuria as a relative contraindication for tranexamic acid. *Br J Haematol* 1995;89(3):663–664.
2. Ghahestani SM, Shakhssalim N. Palliative treatment of intractable hematuria in context of advanced bladder cancer: a systematic review. *Urol J* 2009;6(3):149–156.
3. Abt D, Bywater M, Engeler DS, Schmid HP. Therapeutic options for intractable hematuria in advanced bladder cancer. *Int J Urol* 2013;20(7):651–660.

Chapter 18

Metabolic Acidosis

Joseph Arthur

Classification

- High anion gap metabolic acidosis (HAGMA, mnemonic MUDPILES)—Methanol, Uremia, Diabetic ketoacidosis/alcoholic ketoacidosis/starvation ketoacidosis, Paraldehyde/phenformin/metformin, Iron/isoniazid, Lactic acidosis (cyanide, hydrogen sulfide, carbon monoxide, met hemoglobin), Ethylene glycol, Salicylates
- Non-anion gap metabolic acidosis (NAGMA, also called hyperchloremic acidosis)
  - Gastrointestinal causes—Diarrhea, laxatives, ileostomy, intestinal or pancreatic fistulas or drainage, ureterosigmoidoscopy
  - Renal causes—Renal tubular acidosis, renal failure, hypoaldosteronism, drugs (amiloride, acetazolamide, triamterene, spironolactone, β-blockers)
  - Dilutional acidosis—Due to rapid infusion of bicarbonate-free isotonic saline as seen in volume resuscitation)
  - Ureteral diversion

Symptoms and Signs

- Mainly manifestations related to the underlying cause of the acidosis.

Investigations

See Figure 18.1 for the diagnostic approach to metabolic acidosis.
- First, determine whether it is HAGMA or NAGMA
  - Anion gap (AG) = $Na-[Cl + HCO_3]$
  - Normal AG reference range is generally 9 ± 4 mEq/L, although it may vary from one laboratory to the other.
  - HAGMA = higher than the reference range
  - NAGMA = within the reference range
- For HAGMA, check for the presence of ketones, which indicates ketoacidosis. If ketones are negative, check renal function, lactic acid level, toxicology screen, and osmolar gap (suggests possible methanol or ethylene glycol ingestion).

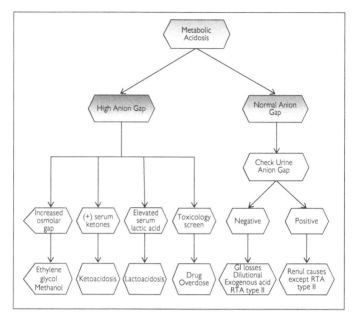

Figure 18.1 Diagnostic approach to metabolic acidosis.

- For NAGMA, first evaluate the history for causes (e.g., diarrhea, medications, intravenous fluids)
  - Check the urine anion gap [(urine sodium + urine potassium) − urine chloride]
  - Positive result indicates renal causes.
  - Negative result indicates gastrointestinal or other causes.

Relevance to the Cancer Palliative Care Setting

- Dysproteinemic states such as multiple myeloma and monoclonal gammopathy may result in NAGMA because they can cause proximal renal tubular acidosis (RTA).
- Lactic acidosis, a known cause of metabolic acidosis, is a rare complication of malignancy.
  - This has been observed more often in hematologic malignancies, but also in solid tumors such as small cell lung cancer, cholangiocarcinoma, breast cancer, gynecologic cancers, and metastasis from unknown primary carcinoma.
  - It is usually associated with high mortality because it is an indication of advanced disease process and high tumor burden.
  - Increased awareness of this complication is important because early initiation of chemotherapy may decrease lactic acidosis and perhaps prolong survival.

Management for Patients with Years of Life Expectancy

- Correct the underlying cause [e.g., diabetic ketoacidosis (DKA), diarrhea, uremia].
- Sodium bicarbonate is generally indicated in NAGMA. The intravenous therapy is indicated in acute situations and the oral form is usually indicated in chronic conditions.
- Use of sodium bicarbonate in HAGMA is controversial. If given, it should be reserved for patients with a pH of <7.10 or in life-threatening cases.
- Hemodialysis may be particularly useful in patients with renal failure.

Management for Patients with Months of Life Expectancy

- This is similar to patients with longer life expectancy.

Management for Patients with Weeks/Days of Life Expectancy

- Patients with advanced cancer who have severe metabolic acidosis (e.g., HCO_3 >16) have a short survival (in terms of hours or days) if the underlying cause cannot be rapidly reversed.
- Emphasis should be placed on interventions aimed at managing distressing symptoms such as vomiting and diarrhea, with the ultimate goal of achieving only short-term benefit.

Recommended Reading

1. de Groot R, Sprenger RA, et al. Type B lactic acidosis in solid malignancies. *Neth J Med* 2011;69(3):120–123.
2. Alguire PC, Epstein PE. Acid-base disorders. MKSAP14. *Medical Knowledge and Self-Assessment Program*. Nephrology: American College of Physicians, Philadelphia, 2011: 19–21.

Chapter 19

Electrolyte Abnormalities (Na, K, Mg)

Masanori Mori

Classification/Causes

- Hyponatremia—Hypertonic, isotonic, hypotonic (hypovolemic, euvolemic, hypervolemic)
- Hypernatremia—Extrarenal water loss, renal water loss, Na overload
- Hypokalemia—Gastrointestinal (GI) losses, renal losses, transcellular shifts
- Hyperkalemia—Decreased renal K excretion, transcellular shifts
- Hypomagnesemia—GI losses, renal losses
- Hypermagnesemia—Increased intake, increase absorption, decreased excretion

Symptoms and Signs

- Hyponatremia—Fatigue, nausea, dizziness, headache, forgetfulness, confusion, lethargy, muscle cramps, gait disturbances, and seizures
- Hypernatremia—Lethargy, weakness, irritability, twitching, seizures, and coma
- Hypokalemia—Nausea, vomiting, anorexia, ileus, muscle cramps, weakness, rhabdomyolysis, myoglobinuria, polyuria, electrocardiogram (ECG) changes, and respiratory failure
- Hyperkalemia—Muscle weakness or paralysis, paresthesias, nausea, palpitations, ECG changes, conduction abnormalities, and arrhythmias
- Hypomagnesemia—Weakness, anorexia, apathy, delirium, coma, hypokalemia, hypocalcemia, metabolic alkalosis, ECG changes, and ventricular arrhythmias
- Hypermagnesemia—Nausea, flushing, headache, weakness, drowsiness, diminished reflexes, hypocalcemia, bradycardia, respiratory paralysis, ECG changes

Investigations

- Hyponatremia—Assess plasma osmolality, volume status, U_{Na}, FE_{Na}, and U_{osm}. See Table 19.1.

Table 19.1 Etiology of Hypotonic Hyponatremia

Type	Key Features	Key Causes
Hypovolemic hyponatremia	U_{Na} >20, FE_{Na} >1%	Renal losses, mineralocorticoid deficiency
	U_{Na} <10, FE_{Na} <1%	Extrarenal losses
Euvolemic hyponatremia	U_{osm} >100	SIADH,* hypothyroidism, glucocorticoid deficiency
	U_{osm} <100	Primary polydipsia, low solute
	U_{osm} variable	Reset osmostat
Hypervolemic hyponatremia	U_{Na} <10, FE_{Na} <1%	Congestive heart failure, cirrhosis, nephrosis
	U_{Na} >20, FE_{Na} >1%	Renal failure

* SIADH, syndrome of inappropriate antidiuretic hormone secretion.

• Hypernatremia—Assess U_{osm}, U_{Na}, and volume status. See Table 19.2.
• Hypokalemia—24-hour U_K and transtubular potassium gradient [TTKG = $(U_K/P_K)/(U_{osm}/P_{osm})$] can differentiate GI ($U_K$ <25 mEq/day, <15 mEq/L, or TTKG <3) versus renal (U_K >30 mEq/day, >15 mEq/L, or TTKG >7) losses; rule out transcellular shifts.
• Hyperkalemia—Assess glomerular filtration rate (GFR); rule out transcellular shift.
• Hypomagnesemia—History can reveal GI versus renal losses most of the time.
• Hypermagnesemia—Check medications, renal function, and GI disorders.

Relevance to the Cancer Palliative Care Setting

• Hyponatremia and hypernatremia may be associated with inpatient mortality.
• Electrolyte abnormalities can be caused by various conditions (e.g., anorexia, vomiting, diarrhea) and comorbidities [e.g., renal insufficiency, paraneoplastic syndrome of inappropriate antidiuretic hormone secretion (SIADH), tumor lysis] associated with cancer and treatment complications. Because of their associated symptom burden and potentially reversible nature, comprehensive assessment and treatment are warranted, if consistent with goals of care.

Table 19.2 Etiology of Hypernatremia

Key Features				Key Causes
U_{osm} >700–800	U_{Na}<25	Extrarenal water loss		GI water loss, insensible loss
		Intracellular osmoles		Seizure, exercise
	U_{Na}>100	Na overload		$NaCl/NaHCO_3$, mineralocorticoids
U_{osm} <700–800	Renal water loss	U_{osm}<300		Complete diabetes insipidus (DI)
		U_{osm} 300–600		Partial DI, osmotic diuresis, loop diuretics

- Mg-containing medications that are routinely used in the palliative care setting should be administered carefully for patients with renal impairment.

Management for Patients with Years of Life Expectancy

- Treat the underlying etiology if possible.
- Hyponatremia
  - Correct with normal or hypertonic saline (rate of increase in Na should not exceed 10–12 mEq/L/day to avoid osmotic demyelination syndrome).
  - SIADH—Free water restrict; hypertonic saline (±loop diuretic); salt tablets; vasopressin receptor antagonist (conivaptan or tolvaptan) if refractory.
  - Hypervolemic hyponatremia—Loop diuretics; vasodilators to increase cardiac output in congestive heart failure (CHF); colloid infusion in cirrhosis; tolvaptan if refractory.
- Hypernatremia—Restore access to water or supply daily requirement of water (>1 L/day); replace free water deficit (rate of decrease in Na should be <0.5 mEq/L/h).
- Hypokalemia—Replete K (KCl 40 mEq PO q4–6h if nonurgent, KCl 10 mEq/h IV if urgent); replete Mg as necessary; avoid K and dextrose-containing solutions.
- Hyperkalemia—Treatment should be initiated promptly. See Table 19.3.
- Hypomagnesemia—Mg repletion (magnesium sulfate 1–2 g, magnesium infusion for severe symptoms, oral magnesium 240–1,000 mg/day for no or minimal symptoms).
- Hypermagnesemia—Discontinue Mg-containing medications (e.g., laxatives, antacids); use intravenous calcium and hemodialysis for emergent treatment.

Table 19.3 Treatment of Hyperkalemia

Treatment	Dose Examples	Comments
Calcium gluconate Calcium chloride	Calcium gluconate 1 g IV (peripheral line) Calcium chloride 0.5–1 g IV (central line)	Transient effect [calcium should be the initial treatment if (+) ECG changes]
Insulin + glucose	Regular insulin 10 U IV + D_{50} W 50 mL	
Sodium bicarbonate	150 mEq + D_5 W 1 L over 2–4 h	
β_2-Agonists	Albuterol 10–20 mg inhaler or 0.5 mg IV	
Kayexalate	30–90 g PO/PR	Decreases total body K
Diuretics	Furosemide ≥ 40 mg IV	
Hemodialysis		

Management for Patients with Months of Life Expectancy

• Management is similar to patients with years of life expectancy, although the appropriateness of aggressive care such as hemodialysis should be discussed.

Management for Patients with Weeks/Days of Life Expectancy

• Electrolyte abnormalities may not be the source of suffering in the terminal phase. Hydration, fluid restriction, or blood work may cause an additional burden. Since aggressive treatment can be distressful, care focusing on comfort is essential.

Recommended Reading

1. Sabatine MS. *Pocket Medicine* (4th ed.). Lippincott Williams & Wilkins, Philadelphia, PA, 2011.

2. Yu ASL, Ahluwalia, GKK. Evaluation and treatment of hypomagnesemia; Agus ZS. Signs and symptoms of magnesium depletion; Agus ZS. Causes and treatment of hypermagnesemia. UpToDate®.

3. Elsayem A, Mori M, Parsons HA, et al. Predictors of inpatient mortality in an acute palliative care unit at a comprehensive cancer center. *Support Care Cancer* 2010;18(1):67–76.

Chapter 20

Hypercalcemia

Kimberson Tanco

Causes

- Malignancy—Most common cause in hospital setting; humoral hypercalcemia of malignancy, osteolytic hypercalcemia, secretion of active vitamin D, ectopic parathyroid hormone (PTH) secretion
- Parathyroid—Primary hyperparathyroidism [the most common cause in the community], familial, lithium-induced release of PTH
- Granulomatous disorder (e.g., sarcoidosis)
- Bone—Increased bone turnover seen in hyperthyroidism, immobilization, thiazides, vitamin A intoxication, hyperparathyroidism, malignancy
- Nephrologic—Renal failure, milk-alkali syndrome, familial hypocalciuric hypercalcemia
- Gastrointestinal—Increased intestinal calcium absorption in vitamin D toxicity, vitamin A toxicity

Symptoms and Signs

- Cardiac—Bradycardia, hypotension, arrhythmia (electrocardiogram changes include short QT, wide T, and prolonged PR)
- Central nervous system (CNS)—Memory loss, mood changes, concentration changes, irritability, delirium, sedation, stupor, coma
- Gastrointestinal—Nausea, vomiting, constipation, anorexia, acute pancreatitis, peptic ulcers
- Nephrologic—Polyuria, polydipsia, dehydration, decreased glomerular filtration, renal insufficiency, nephrolithiasis

Investigations

- Corrected total serum calcium or serum ionized calcium
  - Corrected total serum calcium:
    - In Imperial Units: corrected calcium (mg/dL) = serum calcium + 0.8 × (4 − serum albumin in g/dL)

- In SI Units: corrected calcium (mmol/L) = serum calcium + 0.2 × (40 − serum albumin in g/L)
- Parathyroid hormone-related protein—Levels greater than 12 pmol/L may reflect bisphosphonate resistance
- 1,25(OH)$_2$D$_3$—Elevated in granulomatous disorders such as sarcoidosis and lymphomas
- Other laboratory tests—Serum electrolytes, phosphorus, creatinine, alkaline phosphatase

Relevance to the Cancer Palliative Care Setting

- Hypercalcemia is a metabolic emergency and the most common paraneo-plastic syndrome. Malignancy is the most frequent cause of hypercalcemia in the hospital setting. It is more common in certain cancers, such as squamous cell non-small cell lung cancer, breast cancer, head and neck cancer, myeloma, and renal cell carcinoma.
  - The median survival is approximately 1 month for patients with advanced cancer presenting with hypercalcemia.
  - Hypercalcemia is associated with many common issues in patients with advanced cancer, such as delirium, pain, and constipation.

Management of Patients with Years of Life Expectancy

- Hydration—Key initial step in treating hypercalcemia. Mild hypercalcemia can be corrected by outpatient oral rehydration. Concurrent electrolyte abnormalities may also be present and should be monitored.
- Bisphosphonates [e.g., zoledronic acid, pamidronate, clodronate (Table 20.1)]—Mainstay of treatment; it works by inhibiting osteoclastic bone resorption through osteoclastic apoptosis. Administer parenterally due to

Table 20.1 Common Therapeutic Dosage

- IV or SC hydration—isotonic saline ≥1–3 L/day
- Bisphosphonates
  - Nitrogen-containing
    - Pamidronate 60–90 mg IV
    - Zoledronate 4 mg IV in 50 mL of normal saline over 15 min
  - Non-nitrogen-containing
    - Clodronate 1,500 mg IV or SC single dose or 300 mg IV daily × 7–10 days
- Calcitonin 4–8 IU/kg SC/IM q6–12 h
- Corticosteroids
  - Dexamethasone 4–12 mg/day IV/PO
  - Prednisone 25–75 mg/day IV/PO
- Gallium nitrate 100–200 mg/m^2/day IV over 24 h × 5 days

poor oral bioavailability. Adverse effects include hypocalcemia, nephrotoxicity, osteonecrosis of the jaw, ocular reactions, and acute phase reactions such as fever, myalgias, bone pain flare, and lymphocytopenia.

- Calcitonin—Inhibits bone resorption and renal tubular calcium reabsorption. Subcutaneous administration has an onset of action in 2–4 hours. Continued administration >48 hours leads to tachyphylaxis and diminished effect secondary to downregulation of osteoclastic calcitonin receptors. It is useful when combined with bisphosphonates. Adverse effects include nausea, abdominal pain, flushing, and local site irritation.

- Corticosteroids—Used in hypercalcemia secondary to steroid-responsive tumors such as lymphoma or myeloma. May be an effective adjunct to calcitonin as it prolongs the effective time of treatment of calcitonin.

- RANKL inhibitors (e.g., denosumab, osteoprotegerin)—Interferes with osteoclast recruitment and differentiation. The use is limited by cost.

- Diuretics—No longer recommended due to risks of further volume depletion and electrolyte imbalance.

- Gallium nitrate—Found to be effective in both parathyroid hormone-related protein (PTHrP)-mediated and non-PTHrP-mediated hypercalcemia. Adverse effects include nephrotoxicity, hypophosphatemia, and nausea. It needs a 5 day administration time.

- Treatment of the underlying cause (e.g., antineoplastics in terms of cancer) and discontinuation of hypercalcemia-inducing medications.

Management for Patients with Months of Life Expectancy

- Management is similar to patients with years of life expectancy.

Management for Patients with Weeks/Days of Life Expectancy

- Hypercalcemia is associated with many common issues in patients with advanced cancer, such as delirium, pain, and constipation. Appropriate treatment of hypercalcemia may help improve patients' quality of life.

- Goals of care should guide the overall treatment approach. For patients who are expected to have days of survival, reversal of hypercalcemia may not be necessary.

Recommended Reading

1. Leboff MS, Mikulee KH. Hypercalcemia: Clinical manifestations, pathogenesis, diagnosis, and management. In Favus MJ (ed.). *Primer on the Metabolic Bone Diseases and Disorders of Mineral Metabolism* (5th ed.). American Society for Bone and Mineral Research, Washington, DC, 2003: 225–229.

2. Body JJ. Hypercalcemia of malignancy. *Semin Nephrol* 2004;24:48–54.

3. Clines GA, Guise TA. Hypercalcemia of malignancy and basic research on mechanisms responsible for osteolytic and osteoblastic metastasis to bone. *Endocr Relat Cancer* 2005;12:549–583.

4. Agraharkar M, Dellinger OD, Gangakhedkar AK. Hypercalcemia. Medscape Reference, 2010.

Section V

Gastrointestinal

Chapter 21

Upper and Lower Gastrointestinal Bleeding

Jung Hye Kwon and Kyung Ho Kim

Causes

- Upper gastrointestinal (GI) bleeding (above the ligament of Treitz)
  - Mucosal ulceration (gastritis, or ulceration)
  - Tumor bleeding [esophageal cancer, gastric cancer, lymphoma, gastrointestinal stromal tumor (GIST), and metastasis involving the stomach]
  - Portal hypertension (esophageal or gastric varices)
  - Esophageal tears
- Lower GI bleeding
  - Massive upper gastrointestinal bleeding
  - Diverticular bleeding
  - Angiodysplasia
  - Tumor bleeding (rectal cancer, colon cancer, direct invasion or metastasis of other cancer)
  - Inflammatory bowel disease
  - Postradiation proctitis
  - Rectal or colonic ulceration
- Systemic causes
  - Severe thrombocytopenia
  - Disseminated intravascular coagulation (DIC)
  - Bone marrow failure
  - Drug induced (e.g., bevacizumab)
  - End-stage cirrhosis
  - Advanced hematologic disease

Symptoms and Signs

- Symptoms—Dizziness, palpitation, abdominal pain, emesis, fever, weight loss
- Signs
  - General: Hemodynamic instability including postural changes in heart rate or blood pressure, tachycardia, and recombinant hypotension
  - Upper GI bleeding: Hematemesis, occult blood positive stools, melena

- Lower GI bleeding: Hematochezia, the passage of bright red blood, clots, or maroon stools per rectum, melena or black stools

Investigations

- Upper intestinal bleeding: Complete blood cell count (CBC), coagulation profile [PT with international normalized ratio (INR), activated partial thromboplastin time (aPTT)]
- For comorbidities: Electrolytes and liver function test
- For DIC: FDP, D-dimer, antithrombin III
- Upper intestinal bleeding:
  - Nasogastric aspiration (NGA): Presence of blood or "coffee-ground" appearance, sometimes clear
  - Upper GI endoscopy: Contraindicated in neutropenic patients (absolute neutrophil count $\leq$500/mm^3)
- Lower intestinal bleeding
  - Upper GI endoscopy for massive bleeding
  - Sigmoidoscopy, colonoscopy, and ^{99m}TC-labeled red cell scan
- Obscure origin: Push enteroscopy, video capsule endoscopy, double-balloon enteroscopy, enteroclysis, angiography

Management for Patients with Years of Life Expectancy

- Initial management includes volume resuscitation with crystalloids in addition to packed red blood cells (PRBC) transfusion, along with large bore intravenous access, oxygen supply, and monitoring.
- Upper GI bleed
  - Nasogastric aspiration with lavage may be useful in confirming the source and the briskness of bleeding in patients with suspected upper GI bleeding.
  - Coagulopathy can be corrected with administration of fresh frozen plasma (FFP). To prevent dilutional coagulopathy and keep the international normalized ratio (INR) less than 1.5, 1 unit of FFP for every 4 units of PRBCs can be used.
  - Platelets should be replaced in patients with ongoing GI bleeding when the platelet count is less than 50,000.
  - Initial empiric therapy with a proton pump inhibitor (PPI) is recommended before upper endoscopy in patients with suspected upper GI bleeding.
  - Endoscopy should be performed within 24 hours once the patient has been stabilized hemodynamically to confirm the diagnosis and to treat an identified lesion by endoscopic hemostasis in patients with suspected upper GI bleeding.
  - Endoscopic variceal ligation (EVL) or injection sclerotherapy can be used in patients with cirrhosis or hepatocellular carcinoma, along with somatostatin therapy and prophylactic antibiotic therapy.
  - Balloon tamponade should be used as a temporary measure for a maximum of 24 hours in patients with uncontrollable variceal bleeding awaiting

definitive measure, such as a transjugular intrahepatic portosystemic shunt procedure.

- Lower GI bleed
  - Colonoscopy should be considered to diagnose and treat a bleeding lesion by endoscopic hemostasis in patients with suspected lower GI bleeding.
  - Angiography may be used to diagnose and treat severe bleeding, especially when the bleeding source cannot be identified by upper and lower endoscopy.
  - Patients with massive bleeding that cannot be controlled by endoscopy or angiography may require surgery.
  - Somatostatin or octreotide may be considered in patients with severe ongoing bleeding who are not responsive to endoscopic therapy, intravenous PPI, or both, and are not surgical candidates.

Relevance to the Cancer Palliative Care Setting

- As gastrointestinal bleeding in the cancer patient is often caused by reversible disease such as peptic ulcer or diverticular bleeding, urgent endoscopy should be considered in all patients with a reasonable performance status and life expectancy.
- Surgery may be indicated for a small group of well-selected patients who have failed conservative measures and who are fit for surgery.

Management for Patients with Months of Life Expectancy

- Similar to management for patients with longer life expectancy.
- Angiography with embolization may be used to treat a patient who has recurrent or persistent GI bleed despite endoscopic hemostasis and/or medical therapy.

Management for Patients with Weeks/Days of Life Expectancy

- Invasive measures such as endoscopy, angiography, and surgery may be harmful in these patients, and comfort care should be the priority.
- Conservative care including fluid therapy, blood transfusions, and/or empiric PPI therapy may be the primary modalities in these patients.

Recommended Reading

1. Imbesi JJ, Kurtz RC. A multidisciplinary approach to gastrointestinal bleeding in cancer patients. *J Support Oncol* 2005;3(2):101–110.

2. Yarris JP, Warden CR. Gastrointestinal bleeding in cancer patients. *Emerg Med Clin North Am* 2009;27(3):363–379

3. Pereira J, Phan T. Management of bleeding in patients with advanced cancer. *The Oncologist* 2004;9:561–570.

Chapter 22

Acute and Chronic Diarrhea

Zubia S. Ahmad and Egidio Del Fabbro

Definition

- Three or more unformed stools within 24 hours.
- Diarrhea is often acute and symptoms resolve spontaneously within a few days.
- Diarrhea that persists longer than 3 weeks is considered chronic.

Causes

- Secretory
  - Medications—Senna, dulcolax
  - Infections—Cholera, *Staphylococcus, Bacillis cereus, Clostridium perfringens, Escherichia coli*, rotavirus, norovirus, cytomegalovirus, *Giardia, Cryptococcus, Amoeba*
  - Neuroendocrine tumors—Carcinoid, VIPoma, calcitoninoma, gastrinoma, somatostatinoma
  - Others—Bile salt enteropathy, fatty acid-induced, collagenous colitis, lymphocytic colitis
- Osmotic
  - Malabsorption—Pancreatic insufficiency, celiac disease, lactose intolerance, short bowel syndrome, enteric fistula, bacterial overgrowth
  - Medications—Antacids, antibiotics, colchicine, magnesium citrate, magnesium hydroxide, lactulose, sorbitol
- Inflammatory
  - Infections—*Salmonella, Shigella, Yersinia, Campylobacter, Escherichia coli* (EHEC, EIEC), *Clostridium difficile, Amoeba*
  - Inflammatory—Ulcerative colitis, Crohn's, ischemic, radiation, toxic
  - Medications—Chemotherapy, targeted agents (e.g., erlotinib)
- Motility disorders—Hyperthyroidism, diabetic neuropathy, irritable bowel syndrome (IBS), scleroderma
- Overflow diarrhea

Table 22.1 National Cancer Institute-Common Toxicity Criteria (NCI-CTC) v.4.02	
Grade	Description
1	Increase of <4 stools/day over baseline; mild increase in ostomy output compared to baseline
2	Increase of 4–6 stools/day over baseline; moderate increase in ostomy output compared to baseline
3	Increase of ≥7 stools/day over baseline; incontinence; hospitalization indicated; severe increase in ostomy output compared to baseline; limiting self-care ADL
4	Life-threatening consequences; urgent intervention indicated
5	Death

Symptoms and Signs

- A history may identify potential causes for acute or chronic diarrhea. Inquire about the frequency of bowel movements, consistency of feces, time course of symptoms, and weight loss. Cancer diagnosis and treatments, other medications (e.g., laxatives), dietary habits, and travel history may inform the diagnosis. See Table 22.1 for the grading of diarrhea.
- The physical examination should include vital signs, inspection of oral mucosa and skin turgor, perineum skin integrity, and abdominal examination. A rectal examination may be needed to rule out fecal impaction and to collect a stool sample for studies.

Investigations

- Laboratory tests for patients with diarrhea may include stool cultures, Gram stains, fecal leukocyte count, Clostridium difficile toxin, electrolytes, creatinine, and complete blood count.
- Consider serum levels or empiric treatment of vitamin ADEK deficiencies related to chronic malabsorptive diarrhea.
- Radiographic procedures such as a kidney, ureter, bladder (KUB), and abdominal computed tomography (CT) are indicated if severe constipation, ileus, obstruction, or another mechanical abnormality is suspected.
- Endoscopy may be indicated in rare cases in which diarrhea is persistent and no cause has been identified using less invasive techniques.

Relevance to the Cancer Palliative Care Setting

- Up to 70% of patients with carcinoid syndrome may experience diarrhea. Octreotide reduces diarrhea by inhibiting vasoactive intestinal peptide secretion and increasing water and electrolyte absorption.
- Cancer treatments such as chemotherapy, targeted therapy, bone marrow transplant, abdominal/pelvic radiation, and surgical resection of the

gastrointestinal (GI) tract can contribute to diarrhea in cancer patients. There may be more than one mechanism of diarrhea for some patients.

- Radiation-induced diarrhea—Dose dependent (e.g., >15 Gy to small bowel).
- Alterations in GI motility can also be the result of a celiac plexus block for pain or prior surgeries including gastrectomy or postvagotomy.
- Diarrhea occurs in 7–10% of cancer patients admitted to hospice.

Management of Patients with Years of Life Expectancy

- When possible, treat the underlying cause of diarrhea (see Table 22.2).
- Severe diarrhea not responding to dietary modification and initial therapy, or accompanied by fever, neutropenia, bleeding, cramping, hypotension, and vomiting, requires admission for intravenous fluids, octreotide, and possibly antibiotics.
- The BRAT (bananas, rice, apples, toast) diet may decrease stool frequency in patients with moderate diarrhea. Reduce the intake of dairy products and foods high in fiber or fat.

Table 22.2 Causes and Treatment of Diarrhea in Patients with Cancer

Causes	Description	Treatment
Laxative overuse	Common cause of diarrhea in palliative care	Decrease/stop laxatives
Overflow diarrhea	Fecal impaction secondary to severe constipation	Laxatives, rectal disimpaction
Bacterial infection	Salmonella, Shigella, Campylobacter, C. difficile	Antibiotics
Viral infection	Cytomegalovirus, adenovirus, rotavirus, Norwalk virus, HIV	Supportive care, intravenous fluids
Metastatic carcinoid tumor	Serotonin elevated, secretory diarrhea	Octreotide
Zollinger–Ellison syndrome	Hypergastrinemia	Surgical resection
Postileal resection	Bile salt diarrhea	Cholestyramine
Malabsorption/ steatorrhea	Due to decreased exocrine pancreatic function	Pancreatic enzyme replacement
Chemotherapy-induced diarrhea	Colitis related to mucosal damage	Loperamide, octreotide
Graft-versus-host disease (GVHD)	In addition to diarrhea, acute GVHD of the distal small bowel and colon may present with abdominal pain and intestinal bleeding	Nonabsorbable corticosteroids such as oral budesonide and beclomethasone dipropionate
Pelvic/abdominal radiation	Diarrhea starting the second and third week of radiation	Consider prophylactic lactobacillus
Enteral feeding	Osmotic diarrhea may be due to formula or rate	Adjust type and rate of formula

- *Clostridium difficile* diarrhea—Can occur throughout the disease trajectory, is associated with antibiotic use, is diagnosed by a toxin stool test, and is treated with metronidazole. Oral vancomycin may also be considered as a second line option.
- Chemotherapy-induced diarrhea
  - This is particularly common with irinotecan- and 5-fluorouracil-based regimens, but may also occur with many other chemotherapeutic and targeted agents such as erlotinib.
  - The first line treatment is loperamide 4 mg in the morning and 2 mg after every bout of diarrhea, with a maximum of 16 mg/day. The second line treatment is octreotide.
  - In severe cases, a dose reduction or treatment discontinuation may be needed.
  - Probiotics may reduce chemotherapy- and radiation-induced diarrhea.
- Bone marrow transplant patients with graft-versus-host disease respond to nonabsorbable corticosteroids such as beclomethasone, budesonide, and systemic prednisone.
- Ileal resection in gastric or pancreatic cancer results in poor reabsorption of bile salts causing secretory effects that can be managed with cholestyramine.
- Enteral feeding-related diarrhea—the rate or formula may need to be changed.

Management of Patients with Months of Life Expectancy

- Management of diarrhea similar to those patients with years of life expectancy.
- Dietary modification can reduce symptom burden and oral hydration with clear fluids containing both glucose and electrolytes should be encouraged.
- If oral hydration cannot be tolerated, consider hospitalization for rehydration with intravenous fluids.

Management of Patients with Weeks/Days of Life Expectancy

- Laxative overuse and leakage around fecal impaction are common causes for diarrhea in palliative care patients. They can potentially be easily reversed.
- Patients who are dehydrated and unable to swallow may benefit from intravenous, subcutaneous, or enteral fluids and repletion of electrolytes, providing that death is not imminent and hydration is compatible with the goals of care.
- Symptomatic treatment with opioids and octreotide may be appropriate for some patients.

Recommended Reading

1. Benson AB, Afjani J, Catalano R, et al. Recommended guidelines for the treatment of cancer treatment-induced diarrhea. *J Clin Oncol* 2004;22(4):2918–2926.

2. Gastrointestinal Complications (PDQ®), Health Professional Version. http://www.cancer.gov/cancertopics/pdq/supportivecare/gastrointestinalcomplications/HealthProfessional/page5.

Chapter 23

Bowel Obstruction

Egidio Del Fabbro

Classification and Causes

- Malignant mechanical bowel obstruction (MBO)
  - Mechanism
    - Intraluminal obstruction
    - External compression—peritoneal carcinomatosis
  - Anatomic site
    - Gastric
    - Small bowel
    - Colorectal
  - Complete versus incomplete
- Fecal impaction
- Non-cancer-related bowel obstruction
  - Adhesions, hernias, inflammatory bowel disease, diverticulitis
- Adynamic
  - Pseudoobstruction
  - Ileus

Symptoms and Signs

- Nausea, vomiting, and abdominal pain
- Proximal obstruction is likely to result in greater nausea and vomiting, whereas more distal obstructions may have fewer symptoms and more signs, including distention and air-fluid levels on radiographs.
- Infrequent or no bowel movements and minimal flatus

Investigations

- Plain radiography is useful but may not demonstrate air-fluid levels or other abnormalities even in the presence of obstruction.
- Contrast radiographs (e.g., barium swallow) are useful to distinguish dysmotility and pseudoobstruction from MBO. Small bowel follow-through may be helpful in patients with normal radiographs or low-grade obstruction.

- Computed tomography (CT) scan has high sensitivity and specificity and is often necessary to locate the site of obstruction and to inform decision making regarding surgical or endoscopic management.

Relevance in the Cancer Palliative Care Setting

- MBO affects 3–15% of cancer patients. Patients with gastrointestinal (10–40%) and gynecologic (10–30%) malignancies are at a much higher risk of developing MBO.
- The median life expectancy in operable patients with MBO is approximately 4–6 months. For inoperable patients with MBO, the median survival is approximately 4–6 weeks.

Management of Patients with Years of Life Expectancy

- Hydration, pain and nausea control, and bowel rest represent the main supportive measures for bowel obstruction.
- Surgery—Surgical intervention for the individual patient should be considered if the potential benefits outweigh the risks. Surgical management may include bowel resection, stoma creation, bowel bypass, and adhesiolysis.
  - Factors associated with a poor surgical outcome include peritoneal carcinomatosis, multifocal obstruction, large ascites, hypoalbuminemia, and leukocytosis.
  - Patients with partial small bowel obstruction (SBO) or large bowel obstruction have better outcomes with surgery than those with complete SBO. Synchronous presentation of both stage IV malignancy and bowel obstruction carries a better prognosis than metachronous presentation.

Management of Patients with Months of Life Expectancy

- Supportive measures include metoclopramide (if not complete bowel obstruction) or haloperidol for nausea, opioids for pain, octreotide to reduce secretions, and parenteral fluids for hydration.
- Surgery—Patients with factors associated with poor outcome (e.g., advanced age, malnutrition, poor performance status, multiple levels of occlusion, extraabdominal metastases, refractory ascites, a history of abdominal radiotherapy) and high risk of 30 day mortality should not be offered surgical intervention.
- Stenting can be highly successful (>90%) for isolated lesions in the proximal small bowel or colon and may be a reasonable alternative to surgical intervention for patients who are either inoperable or decline surgery. It can also be used as a "bridge" to surgery, where it is cost effective, and is likely to facilitate single-stage surgery.
- Parenteral nutrition should be considered only in selected patients with operable tumors, with slow-growing tumors (e.g., carcinoid), or who have a

prognosis of at least 3 months. It requires frequent blood tests and monitoring and is associated with an increased risk of infections, thrombosis, hyperglycemia, diarrhea, and liver failure.

- Percutaneous endoscopic venting gastrostomy tube (VGT) placement provides symptom relief in >90% of patients with MBO. G-tube placement remains a potential option even in patients with ascites, peritoneal carcinomatosis, and tumor encasement of the stomach.

Management of Patients with Weeks/Days of Life Expectancy

See Figure 23.1 for management of Malignant Bowel Obstruction.

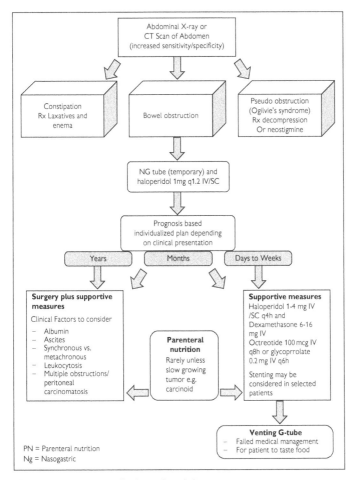

Figure 23.1 Management of malignant bowel obstruction.

- Medical management is preferred in those patients with limited life expectancy.
  - Haloperidol is the drug of choice for nausea and can be given intravenously or subcutaneously. Metoclopramide should be given only in partial bowel obstruction.
  - Opioids intravenously, subcutaneously, or per rectum are usually required for control of pain.
  - Anticholinergics such as hyoscine and glycopyrrolate reduce secretions and are less expensive than octreotide, a synthetic analogue of somatostatin; however, octreotide is superior in reducing nausea and decreasing secretions more rapidly, with doses starting at 300 μg daily.
  - Anticholinergics also have the potential for causing side effects in patients with limited life expectancy, including delirium.
  - Corticosteroids given intravenously (dose range of 6–16 mg dexamethasone) may improve bowel obstruction temporarily.
- In patients who wish to continue taking orally to experience the sensation of taste, a VGT may be considered. A VGT should also be considered in those patients not responding to medical management.
- Nasogastric suctioning should be considered as a temporary measure to decrease a large amount of secretions before the start of specific pharmacologic management to reduce nausea, vomiting, and pain.

Recommended Reading

1. Soriano A, Davis MP. Malignant bowel obstruction: individualized treatment near the end of life. *Cleve Clin J Med* 2011;78:197–206.
2. Henry JC, Pouly S, Sullivan R, et al. A scoring system for the prognosis and treatment of malignant bowel obstruction. *Surgery* 2012;152:747.

Chapter 24

Liver Failure and Hepatitis

Caroline Ha

Classification

- Acuity—Acute hepatitis is <6 months duration. Chronic hepatitis is >6 months duration.
- There are numerous causes of liver failure. Some of the common causes include the following:
  - Cancer—Liver metastases, hepatoma
  - Infections—Hepatitis A/B/C/D/E, Epstein–Barr virus, cytomegalovirus, herpes simplex virus, varicella zoster virus, toxoplasmosis
  - Toxins—Alcoholic liver disease, medications [acetaminophen, nonsteroidal antiinflammatory drugs (NSAIDs), amiodarone, labetalol, statins, phenytoin, valproic acid, fluoroquinolones, amoxicillin/clavulanate, sulfonamides, tetracyclines, isoniazid, azoles, halogen anesthetics, glyburide, propylthiouracil], illicit drugs (cocaine, ecstasy, phencyclidine)
  - Infiltrative—Nonalcoholic fatty liver disease, hemochromatosis, Wilson's disease, glycogen storage disease
  - Autoimmune—Autoimmune hepatitis, primary biliary cirrhosis, primary sclerosing cholangitis
  - Vascular—Ischemic liver, hepatic vein obstruction (Budd–Chiari syndrome), heart failure (congestive liver), venoocclusive disease (hematopoietic stem cell transplant, chemotherapy, oral contraceptives)
  - Cholestasis (see Chapter 25)

Prognosis

- Compensated chronic liver disease—No ascites, hepatic encephalopathy, variceal bleeding, or jaundice; median survival is 12 years. Decompensated liver failure has a median survival of 2 years.
- Child–Pugh classification for chronic liver disease (Table 24.1)
  - Class A—Score 5–6; 1 year survival 95%, 2 year survival 90%
  - Class B—Score 7–9; 1 year survival 80%, 2 year survival 70%
  - Class C—Score ≥10; 1 year survival 45%, 2 year survival 38%
- Model for end-stage liver disease (MELD) score—Estimates the short-term prognosis and is also used to determine eligibility for liver transplantation.

Table 24.1 Child–Pugh Classification			
Scored Item	**1**	**2**	**3**
Serum bilirubin (mg/dL)	<2	2-3	>3
Serum albumin (g/dL)	>3.5	3-3.5	<3
Prothrombin time prolongation (sec) or	0–4	4–6	>6
International normalized ratio (INR)	<1.7	1.7–2.3	>2.3
Ascites	None	Mild	Moderate or severe
Hepatic encephalopathy	None	Grade 1–2	Grade 3–4

The MELD score calculation uses bilirubin, creatinine, and international normalized ratio (INR) in a complex formula.

- Hepatorenal syndrome
  - Type 1—Rapid, severe renal failure; prognosis <10 weeks
  - Type 2—Chronic renal failure, creatinine generally 1.5–2 mg/dL; prognosis <6 months

Symptoms and Signs

- Symptoms—Fatigue, lethargy, weakness, nausea, poor appetite, jaundice, dark urine, itching, abdominal or liver capsule pain, back pain, bloating, easy bleeding and bruising
- Signs—Scleral icterus, jaundice, hepatomegaly, hepatic tenderness, spider angiomata, palmar erythema, edema, ascites, muscle wasting, weight loss, asterixis, altered mental status, stupor or coma, gynecomastia, testicular atrophy, menstrual irregularities, and ecchymoses

Investigations

- Laboratory tests are used to assess liver function and identify potential causes.
  - Serum alanine and aspartate aminotransferases (ALT and AST), alkaline phosphatase, direct and total serum bilirubin, albumin, and prothrombin time/INR should be measured.
  - Serum ammonia should be assessed in patients with altered mental status.
  - If ascites is present, ascitic fluid can be checked for white blood count, albumin, protein, and cytology.
  - Typical tests include hepatitis B surface antigen, IgM anti-hepatitis B core (anti-HBc), anti-hepatitis C virus (anti-HCV), IgM anti-hepatitis A virus (anti-HAV), monospot, ceruloplasmin, antinuclear antibody (ANA), peripheral antinuclear cytoplasmic antibody (P-ANCA), and smooth muscle antibody (SMA).
- Diagnostic imaging—Ultrasound and computed tomography (CT) are both highly sensitive in detecting biliary dilatation and can be utilized for patients

with suspected obstructive jaundice. They can also assess ascites. Endoscopic retrograde cholangiopancreatography (ERCP) and magnetic resonance cholangiopancreatography (MRCP) are useful for visualizing the biliary tree for obstruction.

- Other tests—Liver biopsy remains the gold standard for diagnosis, grading, and staging of chronic hepatitis; in acute hepatitis, biopsy is reserved for diagnoses that remain uncertain after other tests.

Relevance to the Cancer Palliative Care Setting

- Chronic hepatitis increases the risk of developing hepatocellular carcinoma; likewise, malignant biliary obstruction, hepatic metastases, or cancer therapy can precipitate liver failure.
- Chemotherapy may reactivate hepatitis B. Thus, patients with hematologic malignancies (and some solid tumors) starting intensive chemotherapy should be screened for hepatitis surface antigen prior to treatment initiation and be given lamivudine prophylaxis if surface antigen is positive until at least 3 months after the completion of chemotherapy.
- Many drugs are metabolized in the liver; severe hepatic insufficiency can thus result in drug accumulation. The volume of distribution can be altered by decreased albumin. Failure to adjust medication dosing in liver failure can heighten the risk of adverse effects.
- Liver failure and hepatitis both cause significant symptom burden for cancer patients, and may even be the life-limiting factor in some cases.

Management for Patients with Years of Life Expectancy

- Medication management—Dosages may need adjustment for hepatic insufficiency. NSAIDs can increase the risk of bleeding, gastritis, and renal failure, and should be avoided in favor of acetaminophen. Recommendations based on pharmacokinetics for selected medications are presented in Table 24.2.
- Lifestyle recommendations—Patients should eat a balanced diet including normal amounts of protein, but should avoid consuming large amounts of protein in one meal to decrease the risk of developing encephalopathy. Increased physical activity or therapy can be used to combat deconditioning and muscle wasting. Stop alcohol intake.
- Immunizations—Vaccinations against hepatitis A, hepatitis B, influenza, and pneumococcus are recommended for patients with liver disease.
- Ascites management—Diuretics such as spironolactone and furosemide are the first-line treatments in nonmalignant ascites. Evidence for efficacy in malignant ascites is lacking; however, patients with portal hypertension (serum-ascites albumin gradient, or SAAG, >1.1) may still be given a trial. Intermittent paracentesis of 4–6 L is considered safe and effective.
- Hepatic encephalopathy may be triggered by infections, metabolic derangements, gastrointestinal bleeding, or constipation. Treatment primarily

Table 24.2 Selected Medication Adjustments in Hepatic Failure

Class	Medication	Recommendation
Analgesics	Fentanyl	No adjustment needed.
	Methadone	No adjustment needed in mild to moderate disease; caution in severe disease.
	Acetaminophen	Reduce maximum daily dose to <2 g.
	Hydromorphone	Reduce dose; prolong intervals only in severe disease.
	Morphine Oxycodone	Reduce dose and/or prolong intervals.
	Tramadol Codeine Hydrocodone	Efficacy not well evaluated; analgesia requires liver metabolism. Tramadol doses should be reduced. Hydrocodone doses are limited by acetaminophen content.
Sedatives	Lorazepam Temazepam	No adjustment needed.
	Oxazepam	No adjustment needed in mild to moderate disease; caution in severe disease.
	Midazolam	Reduce dose.
	Diazepam	Caution; half-life can double in cirrhosis.
	Clonazepam	Avoid unless at end of life.
Antiemetics	Metoclopramide	No adjustment needed.
	Ondansetron	Reduce maximum daily dose to 8 mg.

involves identifying and treating the precipitating event, and pharmacologic support can be provided with lactulose or rifaximin. The goal with lactulose is to produce three to five bowel movements per day.

- Esophagogastric varices are diagnosed by esophagogastroduodenoscopy (EGD). Varices can be medically managed with nonselective β-blockers or through procedures such as endoscopic variceal ligation or sclerotherapy. If bleeding is refractory, transjugular intrahepatic portosystemic shunting (TIPS) or liver transplantation may be considered.
- Chronic hepatitis—Pegylated interferon can be used to treat chronic hepatitis B. Antiviral agents used for hepatitis B include lamivudine, adefovir, tenofovir, telbivudine, and entacavir. Hepatitis C is treated with a combination of pegylated interferon and ribavirin. Telaprevir and beceprevir can also be used for hepatitis C. Autoimmune hepatitis is treated with glucocorticoids, with or without azathioprine.
- Biliary obstruction—See Chapter 25.

Management for Patients with Months of Life Expectancy

- Medication management is similar to patients with years of life expectancy.
- Ascites management—For patients requiring frequent paracentesis, intraperitoneal drain or shunt placement can be considered to decrease the

frequency of hospital or clinic visits. If a drainage catheter is used, tunneled catheters are preferred over pigtail catheters, which are more prone to leakage, infection, occlusion, and dislodgement. Most patients with malignant ascites do not have portal hypertension and thus do not benefit from TIPS. Peritovenous shunts have a success rate of <50% in malignant ascites and involve a higher risk procedure than drainage catheter placement.

- Hepatic encephalopathy is not uncommon; management includes lactulose or rifamixin as well as treating any precipitating factors such as infection or dehydration. Advance care planning should be discussed, and patients' preferences regarding hospitalization and resuscitation should be clarified.

Management for Patients with Weeks/Days of Life Expectancy

- Medications or treatments that are no longer beneficial to the patient should be discontinued. Medication doses may need to be reduced further as the patient declines.
- Consider palliative paracenteses in patients with symptomatic ascites who do not already have a drain or shunt.
- Patients may be coagulopathic; avoid venipuncture when possible, as severe ecchymosis or oozing from venipuncture sites can be distressing to the patient and family.

Recommended Reading

1. Ghany M, Hoofnagle JH. Approach to the patient with liver disease. In Longo DL, Fauci AS, Kasper DL, et al. (eds.). *Harrison's Principles of Internal Medicine* (18th ed.). McGraw-Hill Professional, New York, 2011: 2520–2527.

2. Dolan B, Arnold R. Prognosis in decompensated liver failure. Fast Facts and Concepts. September 2007; 189. Available at http://www.eperc.mcw.edu/EPERC/FastFactsIndex/ff_189.htm. Accessed May 20, 2013.

3. Bacon BR. Cirrhosis and its complications. In Longo DL, Fauci AS, Kasper DL, et al. (eds.). *Harrison's Principles of Internal Medicine* (18th ed.). McGraw-Hill Professional, New York, 2011: 2592–2602.

4. Rhee C, Broadbent AM. Palliation and liver failure: palliative medications dosage guidelines. *J Pall Med* 2007;10:677–685.

5. Gulcap R, Dutcher J. Oncologic emergencies. In Longo DL, Fauci AS, Kasper DL, et al. (eds.). *Harrison's Principles of Internal Medicine* (18th ed.). McGraw-Hill Professional, New York, 2011: 2268–2669.

Chapter 25

Biliary Obstruction

Marvin O. Delgado-Guay

Differential Diagnosis/Causes

- Extrahepatic
  - Malignant—Pancreatic cancer, ampullary cancer, cholangiocarcinoma, gallbladder cancer, malignant involvement of the porta hepatis lymph nodes
  - Benign—Choledocholithiasis, primary sclerosing cholangitis, chronic pancreatitis, acquired immunodeficiency syndrome (AIDS) cholangiopathy
- Intrahepatic
  - Viral hepatitis
  - Drug toxicity
    - Pure cholestasis—Anabolic and contraceptive steroids
    - Mixed cholestasis/hepatitis—Chlorpromazine, erythromycin estolate
    - Chronic cholestasis—Chlorpromazine and prochlorperazine
  - Alcoholic hepatitis
  - Primary biliary cirrhosis
  - Primary sclerosing cholangitis
  - Vanishing bile duct syndrome (chronic rejection of liver transplants)
  - Sarcoidosis
  - Inherited disorders—Benign recurrent cholestasis, progressive intrahepatic familial cholestasis, Gilbert's syndrome, Crigler–Najjar syndrome types 1 and 2, Dubin–Johnson syndrome, Rotor syndrome, Alagille syndrome
  - Cholestasis of pregnancy
  - Total parenteral nutrition
  - Nonhepatobiliary sepsis
  - Benign postoperative cholestasis
  - Paraneoplastic syndrome

Signs and Symptoms

- Biliary obstruction in patients with unresectable hepatobiliary cancer is frequently associated with pruritus, anorexia, cholangitis, or hyperbilirubinemia.
- Choledocholithiasis is the most common cause of nonmalignant extrahepatic cholestasis. The clinical presentation can range from mild right upper quadrant discomfort with only minimal elevations of the enzyme tests to ascending cholangitis with jaundice, sepsis, and circulatory collapse. Choledocholithiasis is usually associated with an elevation of the serum alkaline phosphatase out of

proportion to the aminotransferases, although elevation of aminotransferases to greater than 1,000 international unit/L may be seen early in the course.

Investigations

- The first step in evaluating patients whose liver function test (LFT) pattern predominantly reflects cholestasis (i.e, elevated bilirubin, elevated alkaline phosphatase) is to determine whether the cholestasis is due to an intrahepatic or extrahepatic cause.
- A reasonable step is to obtain right upper quadrant ultrasonography. The absence of biliary dilatation suggests intrahepatic cholestasis, whereas the presence of biliary dilatation indicates extrahepatic cholestasis. False-negative results occur in patients with partial obstruction of the bile duct or in patients with cirrhosis or primary sclerosing cholangitis where scarring prevents the intrahepatic ducts from dilating.
- Extrahepatic cholestasis: Computer tomography (CT) is better than ultrasonography for assessing the head of the pancreas and for identifying choledocholithiasis in the distal bile duct, particularly when the ducts are not dilated.
- Magnetic resonance cholangiopancreatography (MRCP) is a noninvasive technique for imaging the bile and pancreatic ducts that may replace endoscopic retrograde cholangiopancreatography (ERCP) as the initial diagnostic test in cases in which the need for intervention is felt to be small.
- ERCP is the gold standard for identifying choledocholithiasis. In addition to its diagnostic capabilities, ERCP allows for therapeutic interventions including the removal of bile duct stones and the placement of a stent.
- Delirium may occur in the setting of severe hepatic failure. Patients may also experience other symptoms including pruritus and abdominal pain.

Relevance in the Cancer Palliative Care Setting

- Malignant causes of extrahepatic cholestasis include pancreatic, gallbladder, ampullary, and cholangiocarcinoma. The last is most commonly associated with primary sclerosing cholangitis (PSC). Hilar lymphadenopathy due to metastases from other cancers (e.g., breast, colon) may also cause obstruction of the extrahepatic biliary tree.
- Other causes of intrahepatic cholestasis in cancer patients include total parenteral nutrition, nonhepatobiliary sepsis, benign postoperative cholestasis, and a paraneoplastic syndrome (Stauffer's syndrome) associated with various malignancies, such as renal cell carcinoma, Hodgkin's lymphoma, medullary thyroid cancer, renal sarcoma, T cell lymphoma, prostate cancer, and several gastrointestinal malignancies.
- Cancer patients with severe hyperbilirubinemia may not be eligible to receive systemic cancer therapies that are metabolized or excreted by the liver.

Biliary drainage may be needed to reduce the bilirubin concentration to an acceptable level first.

• Prolonged jaundice is particularly serious because it can result in malabsorption and hepatic and renal dysfunction.

Management of Patients with Years of Life Expectancy

• Discontinue any medications that potentially can cause biliary obstruction.
• Biliary obstruction is suspected if cholelithiasis or choledocholithiasis is present, there is bile duct dilation, and there is elevation of liver enzymes. ERCP with sphincterotomy has been shown to lower morbidity and mortality in these patients, significantly reducing rates of cholangitis and biliary sepsis.
• ERCP is recommended in patients with evidence of gallstone pancreatitis and suspected biliary obstruction.
• Biliary obstruction can be divided into "low" and "high" bile duct obstruction.
  • Low bile duct obstruction occurs below the usual insertion of the cystic duct. Patients with low bile duct obstruction can have complete drainage of the entire biliary system by a single, well-placed catheter or stent. When possible, these patients are best treated endoscopically, because a stent may allow complete drainage without the nuisance of an external catheter. Endoscopic stents used to treat low bile duct obstruction may be crafted of plastic or self-expanding metal. In unresectable malignancies, metallic stents are favored because they offer a longer mean patency (6–10 months versus 3–6 months for plastic stents).
  • High bile duct obstruction occurs above the cystic duct insertion. High bile duct obstruction is best treated percutaneously, because a specific duct can be targeted to maximize functional liver drainage based on preprocedure imaging. High bile duct isolation is complicated. A clear understanding of the goal of drainage and the patient's treatment plan and prognosis is extremely important.
• Percutaneous transhepatic biliary stenting with metallic stents is an established palliative modality to relieve malignant biliary obstruction. The majority of groups have reported a 95–100% technical success rate in dilated bile ducts and 75% in nondilated bile ducts, with satisfactory biliary decompression and symptom relief in 88–96% of cases.
• Biliary-enteric surgical bypass may be considered in selected patients if the above procedures failed.
• In addition to procedures for relief of biliary obstruction, cholestyramine 4–8 g PO BID, colestipol 2–8 g PO BID, and rifampin 150–300 mg PO BID may be used to reduce pruritus associated with cholestasis.

Management of Patients with Months of Life Expectancy

- Management is similar to patients with years of life expectancy.

Management of Patients with Days to weeks of Life Expectancy

- Management should be guided by goals of care and symptom burden. On the one hand, a procedure may be indicated if the patient has weeks of life expectancy and severe pruritus is present. On the other hand, jaundice itself is not an indication of biliary drainage. Any procedure may have complications, and catheters require maintenance and adjustments to lifestyle that may be difficult to justify in an otherwise asymptomatic patient.
- Active measures to treat pruritus and abdominal pain are recommended.

Recommended Reading

1. Brountzos EN, Ptochis N, Panagiotou I, et al. A survival analysis of patients with malignant biliary strictures treated by percutaneous metallic stenting. *Cardiovasc Intervent Radiol* 2007;30:66–73.

2. Garcarek J, Kurcz J, Guzi ski M, Janczak D, Sasiadek M. Ten years single center experience in percutaneous transhepatic decompression of biliary tree in patients with malignant obstructive jaundice. *Adv Clin Exp Med* 2012;21(5):621–632.

3. Yao LQ, Tang CW, Zheng YY, Feng WM, Huang SX, Bao Y. Percutaneous transhepatic biliary stenting vs. surgical bypass in advanced malignant biliary obstruction: cost-effectiveness analysis. *Hepato-Gastroenterology* 2013;60:42–45.

4. Sut M, Kennedy R, McNamee J, Collins A, Clements B. Long-term results of percutaneous transhepatic cholangiographic drainage for palliation of malignant biliary obstruction. *J Palliat Med* 2010;13:1311–1313.

Chapter 26

Pancreatitis

Marvin O. Delgado-Guay

Introduction

- Acute pancreatitis is an acute or relapsing inflammatory process that may also involve peripancreatic tissues and other organs.
- Although most cases are self-limited, approximately 15% of patients develop significant pancreatic necrosis and organ compromise. Patients with multi-organ involvement and failure almost always have necrosis in 30–50% of the gland and a high mortality rate.

Causes

- Obstructive—Gallstones (45% in general population), pancreas divisum, choledochocele, tumors (e.g., intraductal papillary mucinous neoplasms)
- Iatrogenic—Postendoscopic retrograde cholangiopancreatography
- Toxins/drugs—Alcohol (35% in the general population), azathioprine, sulfa drugs, aminosalicylates, metronidazole, pentamidine, didanosine
- Metabolic—Hypercalcemia, hyperlipidemia
- Infectious—Parasites (*Toxoplasma, Cryptosporidium, Ascaris lumbricoides*), viral (cytomegalovirus, Epstein–Barr virus)
- Vascular—Vasculitis, ischemia

Symptoms and Signs

- Manifestations of acute pancreatitis include sudden onset of epigastric pain, often radiating to the back, often accompanied by nausea, vomiting, fever, and tachycardia.
- Manifestations of chronic pancreatitis include abdominal pain, malabsorption, and diabetes mellitus.
- The physical examination shows epigastric tenderness, abdominal distention, hypoactive bowel sounds, and occasional guarding.

Investigations

- Check the complete blood count (CBC) and differential, electrolytes, blood urea nitrogen (BUN), creatinine (Cr), glucose, aspartate aminotransferase

(AST), alanine aminotransferase (ALT), alkaline phosphatase (ALP), bilirubin, lactate dehydrogenase (LDH), and calcium.

- The diagnosis of acute pancreatitis is made primarily through clinical evaluation and detection of elevated serum concentrations of amylase and lipase (at least three times the normal limit).

- Hyperamylasemia may also be caused by disorders of other organs that produce amylase such as the salivary glands or fallopian tubes and by a perforated ulcer, intestinal ischemia, or chronic renal insufficiency. Detection of an elevated serum lipase is more specific for acute pancreatitis but may be an incidental finding in asymptomatic patients.

- A contrast-enhanced computed tomography (CT) scan is the most specific test and in some cases can differentiate between edematous, interstitial pancreatitis and severe necrotizing pancreatitis. Common findings on CT scan in acute pancreatitis include an enlargement or irregular contour of the gland, peripancreatic inflammation, and fluid collections. Abdominal magnetic resonance imaging (MRI) may be an alternative in patients with hypersensitivity to contrast media.

- Abdominal ultrasonography can be used to detect cholelithiasis in patients with suspected gallstone pancreatitis.

- Magnetic resonance cholangiopancreatography (MRCP), endoscopic ultrasound, and endoscopic retrograde cholangiopancreatography (ERCP) may help to evaluate the patient for the possibility of tumors in recurrent or unexplained pancreatitis.

- Ranson criteria (Table 26.1) remain the most used prognostic scoring system while APACHE is the more complex. Neither should substitute for close clinical judgment of the individual patient.

Table 26.1 Ranson Criteria to Predict Severity of Acute Pancreatitis

0 hours	
Age	>55
White blood cell count	>16,000/mm^3
Blood glucose	>200 mg/dL (11.1 mmol/L)
Lactate dehydrogenase	>350 U/L
Aspartate aminotransferase (AST)	>250 U/L
48 hours	
Hematocrit	Fall by ≥10%
Blood urea nitrogen	Increase by ≥5 mg/dL (1.8 mmol/L) despite fluids
Serum calcium	<8 mg/dL (2 mmol/L)
pO$_2$	<60 mmHg
Base deficit	>4 MEq/L
Fluid sequestration	>6,000 mL

The presence of one to three criteria represents mild pancreatitis; the mortality rate rises significantly with four or more criteria.

Adapted from Ranson, JHC, Rifkind, KM, Roses, DF, et al. Prognostic signs and the role of operative management in acute pancreatitis. *Surg Gynecol Obstet* 1974;139:69.

- A diagnosis of chronic pancreatitis is made by imaging that shows pancreatic calcifications and ductal and parenchymal changes of the pancreas or biochemical tests that show impaired pancreatic function.

Relevance in the Cancer Palliative Care Setting

- Pancreatic tumors should be excluded in the presence of acute pancreatitis of undetermined etiology.
- The exact mechanism whereby a tumor causes acute pancreatitis is unclear. It may be due to obstruction of the pancreatic duct, ischemia secondary to vascular occlusion, or activation of pancreatic enzymes by tumor cells.
- Acute pancreatitis may occur in 3–5% of patients after diagnostic/therapeutic ERCP.
- Hypercalcemia, a common paraneoplastic manifestation, can result in acute pancreatitis by activating trypsinogen within the pancreas and/or calcium deposits in the pancreatic duct.

Management of Patients with Years of Life Expectancy

- Mild acute interstitial pancreatitis usually resolves in a few days and does not result in organ dysfunction. Management consists of supportive measures, including bowel rest (nothing by mouth), intravenous fluid replacement, and narcotics for pain control.
- In patients with severe acute pancreatitis whose condition is not improving or who continue to have fever after 3–5 days, a contrast-enhanced CT scan should be performed to evaluate for necrosis.
  - Prophylactic antibiotic therapy in patients with acute pancreatitis should be limited to those patients with necrotizing pancreatitis (mortality 10–30%).
  - Patients with severe pancreatitis often have prolonged hospitalizations with the inability to take food or liquids by mouth. Recent evidence suggests that early nasojejunal feeding may lower morbidity, particularly infectious complications, when compared with intravenous nutrition. This has not been studied in patients with pancreatitis and advanced or terminal cancer.
- Biliary obstruction is suspected if cholelithiasis or choledocholithiasis is present, there is bile duct dilation, and there is elevation of liver enzymes. ERCP with sphincterotomy has been shown to lower morbidity and mortality in these patients, significantly reducing rates of cholangitis and biliary sepsis.
- Treatment of chronic pancreatitis includes pain control by medical, endoscopic, or surgical methods; pancreatic enzyme supplementation for malabsorption; and careful glucose control for diabetes mellitus.
- Pancreatitis may also lead to splenic vein thrombosis with subsequent gastric varices and bleeding. Some patients with severe pancreatitis and significant necrosis may develop diabetes mellitus.

- Pancreatic pseudocysts (cysts of pancreatic juice that have a fibrous, non-epithelial lining that occurs around the gland) are the most common complication of acute pancreatitis. Symptomatic pseudocysts are treated with percutaneous drainage or endoscopic or surgical drainage via the stomach or duodenum. A patient with an infected pseudocyst (pancreatic abscess) presents with worsening abdominal pain, fever, and an increasing leukocyte count. Treatment is usually percutaneous or surgical drainage and antibiotics.

Management of Patients with Months of Life Expectancy

- Similar to management for patients with years of life expectancy.

Management of Patients with Weeks to Days of Life Expectancy

- Similar to management for patients with years of life expectancy; however, invasive procedures may be minimized if the potential risks outweigh the benefits.
- Supportive measures such as opioids for pain control, mouth care, and bowel rest are key. Consider intravenous or subcutaneous hydration depending on the setting, and maximize antiemetics.

Recommended Reading

1. Swaroop VS, Chari ST, Clain JE. Severe acute pancreatitis. *JAMA* 2004;291:2865.
2. Heinrich S, Schäfer M, Rousson V, Clavien PA. Evidence-based treatment of acute pancreatitis: a look at established paradigms. *Ann Surg* 2006;243:154.

Section VI

Hematologic Disorders

Chapter 27

Anemia

Daniel E. Epner

Classification

- Bleeding: Gastrointestinal tract, hemoptysis, vascular erosion by tumor (for instance head and neck)
- Marrow replacement by tumor, infection, or hematologic malignancy: Leukoerythroblastic picture [teardrop red blood cells (RBCs), nucleated RBCs, early white blood cell precursors, or abnormalities in platelet shape]
- Marrow suppression by chemotherapy: Leukocytes and platelets are also usually reduced.
- Iron, folate, or B_{12} deficiency
- Hemolysis
- Anemia of inflammation ("chronic disease")

Symptoms and Signs

- Symptoms—Fatigue, shortness of breath, chest pain, headache, syncope, vertigo, abnormal menstruation in females
- Signs—Tachycardia, tachypnea, hypotension (if severe of acute onset), pale skin, jaundice (if hemolysis)

Investigations

- Complete blood count with indices [white blood cells (WBCs) and platelet counts], reticulocyte index (reticulocyte count corrected for degree of anemia)
- Peripheral blood smear to show evidence of marrow infiltration by tumor or infection, intravascular hemolysis
- Chemistry panel: Total and indirect bilirubin, lactate dehydrogenase (LDH)
- Selected special tests: Iron studies (iron, total iron binding capacity, ferritin); folate, B_{12} levels; haptoglobin, screening studies for disseminated intravascular coagulation (DIC), Coombs test (Table 27.1)

Table 27.1 Common Causes of Anemia in Cancer Patients and Associated Laboratory Findings

Diagnosis	Laboratory Findings
Bleeding	↑ RI
Iron deficiency	↓ Iron and ferritin, ↑ TIBC, ↓ RI, ↓ MCV
B_{12} or folate deficiency	↓ B_{12} or folate, ↓ RI, ↑ MCV
Marrow suppression by chemotherapy or radiation	↓ WBCs, ↓ platelet count
Hemolysis	↓ Haptoglobin, ↑ indirect bilirubin, ↑ RI, ↑ LDH, fragmented RBCs, possibly + DIC panel, + Coombs test
Marrow infiltration by tumor or infection	Myelophthisic smear: tear drops, nucleated RBCs, large platelets
Cancer-associated inflammation	Normal MCV and other laboratory findings

Abbreviations: DIC, disseminated intravascular coagulation; LDH, lactate dehydrogenase; MCV, mean corpuscular volume; RBCs, red blood cells; RI, reticulocyte index; TIBC, total iron binding capacity; WBCs, white blood cells.

Relevance to the Cancer Palliative Care Setting

- Anemia is seen in almost all cancer patients, either as a result of the cancer itself, complications of cancer, or cancer treatment.
- The potential risks and benefits of evaluating and treating anemia in cancer patients based on their stage of illness, curability, potential for life prolongation, and potential for palliation should be considered.
- A more aggressive approach is appropriate for patients who are curable or early in their course of illness. Anemia is often resolvable or even self-limited in patients who are undergoing treatment with curative intent, whereas it may have less practical importance to patients who are in their final days of life.

Management for Patients with Years of Life Expectancy

- Transfusions are generally provided for Hb <8.0 g/dL. For patients with significant cardiovascular or pulmonary diseases, transfusion may be indicated for Hb <9.0 g/dL.
- Bleeding
  - Transfusion: RBCs, plasma for coagulopathy, platelets for thrombocytopenia if the patient does not have antiplatelet antibodies and has experienced appropriate increment after previous platelet transfusions.
  - Surgery to address acute bleeding from the gastrointestinal tract, lungs, head and neck, or other site.
  - Other procedures to address acute or subacute blood loss: Endoscopic gastroduodenoscopy (EGD) to treat bleeding varices or ulcer; colonoscopy

to address polyp, arteriovenous malformation, or malignant ulcer; bronchoscopy to cauterize, remove, or ablate endobronchial lesion.

- Marrow replacement by tumor or infection:
  - Hormone therapy for prostate cancer or receptor-positive breast cancer.
  - Chemotherapy for responsive tumors, such as hematologic malignancies, breast cancer, germ cell neoplasms (such as testicular cancer), high-grade neuroendocrine malignancies (such as small cell lung cancer), selected sarcomas (such as osteogenic and Ewings).
  - Antimicrobials for fungal infection, mycobacterial infection, or other opportunistic infections in heavily treated patients, such as those undergoing marrow or stem cell transplantation for hematologic malignancy.
  - Bone seeking radionuclide in selected patients with widespread bone metastases (may also require transfusions).
  - Bisphosphonate for widespread metastases, especially breast and prostate cancer.
- Marrow suppression by chemotherapy
  - Chemotherapy holiday to permit marrow recovery.
  - Recombinant erythropoietin may promote tumor growth, thromboembolism, and other side effects and should be used rarely, and not for patients treated with curative intent.

Management for Patients with Months of Life Expectancy

- The general approach is similar to that for patients with years to live. However, providers and patients should carefully consider potential risks and benefits of any intervention and pursue only those likely to appreciably improve the quality of life. Later lines of salvage chemotherapy offer diminishing returns, especially for patients with chemoresistant tumors, such as the majority of solid tumors. Many patients will choose to discontinue chemotherapy. Many patients will also stop transfusions, especially if they are required on a frequent basis or require the patient to travel a long distance to the clinic or hospital.

Management for Patients with Weeks/Days of Life Expectancy

- At the end of life, the focus shifts entirely to comfort and dignity. Minimize frequent blood work and other diagnostic tests.
- Many patients enter home hospice programs and typically forego transfusions, intravenous antibiotics, chemotherapy, radiation, or invasive procedures and opt instead to spend as much time as possible with loved ones at home.

Recommended Reading

1. Wintrobe MW, Greer JP. *Wintrobe's Clinical Hematology, 2009*. Lippincott Williams & Wilkins, Philadelphia, 2009.

2. NCCN Clinical Practice Guidelines in Oncology, Cancer- and Chemotherapy-Induced Anemia, version 1.2013. National Comprehensive Cancer Network, NCCN.org.

Chapter 28

Neutropenia

Meiko Kuriya

Causes

- Intrinsic disorders of proliferation and maturation of myeloid and stem cells
  - Acquired disorders of myeloid or stem cells—leukemias, myelodysplastic syndrome (MDS), aplastic anemia, myelofibrosis, and metastasis
  - Congenital
  - Vitamin B_{12} or folate deficiency
- Secondary neutropenia caused by factors extrinsic to bone marrow myeloid cells
  - Infection—Viral, bacterial, protozoan, fungal
  - Drug induced—Chemotherapy, antibiotics, antiepileptics, and others
  - Radiation therapy
  - Immune induced—Alloimmune, autoimmune
  - Hypersplenism

Signs and Symptoms

- Patients with neutropenia may not experience any specific symptoms.
- However, these patients are at an increased risk of overwhelming sepsis secondary to immunosuppression. Because of the lack of an ability to mount an immune response, fever may sometimes be the only manifestation of a serious infection in neutropenic patients. Thus, patients who are at risk of neutropenia (e.g., 1–2 weeks postchemotherapy) should be educated on checking their body temperature if they feel feverish. Once a fever is confirmed, they should get blood work done immediately to assess the neutrophil count, with prompt initiation of antibiotics if febrile neutropenia is present.
- Febrile neutropenia is an absolute neutrophil count (ANC) <500/µL (or <1,000 and expected to decrease further) plus fever >38°C (100.4°F).
- A history and physical examination should assess for potential foci of infection in patients with febrile neutropenia. Specifically, the physical examination may include assessing for skin rash, catheter insertion sites, oropharynx, perirectal/genital area, chest, costovertebral angle tenderness, and neck stiffness.

Investigations

- Laboratory work—Complete blood count (CBC) with differential, electrolytes, blood urea nitrogen/creatinine (BUN/Cr), liver function test, urinalysis
- Other culture specimens should be obtained as clinically indicated, and may include sputum, urine, indwelling catheter insertion site, skin, stool, and cerebrospinal fluid.
- Image—Chest x-ray, computed tomography/magnetic resonance imaging (CT/MRI) of the central nervous system (CNS), sinus, chest or abdomen/pelvis if appropriate.
- Bone marrow biopsy may be needed to examine specific causes of neutropenia.

Relevance to the Cancer Palliative Care Setting

- Neutropenia is most commonly due to systemic cancer therapy in the oncology setting. Sometimes, malignancies may also result in marrow replacement/hypoplasia resulting in neutropenia.
- Febrile neutropenia is a common life-threatening emergency.
- Some of the analgesic agents such as acetaminophen, nonsteroidal antiinflammatory drugs (NSAIDs), and steroids may mask fever, which could potentially delay the detection of a serious infection in an neutropenic individual. Cancer patients with or at risk of neutropenia may still take these medications sparingly, providing that they record their body temperature before each dose.
- Neutropenic patients are generally asked to avoid consuming fresh fruits and vegetables, unpasteurized dairy products, and raw eggs or meats. They should also minimize contact with fresh flowers/plants and any individuals with obvious active infections. They should also maintain good personal hygiene and wash their hands often.

Management for Patients with Years of Life Expectancy

- Treat the etiology of neutropenia if clinically indicated (e.g., discontinue responsible drugs).
- Patients with neutropenia alone and no fever do not require any antibiotic treatments. For selected patients at risk of developing recurrent neutropenia with chemotherapy administration, granulocyte colony-stimulating factor (G-CSF) may be indicated for prophylaxis.
- Treatment of febrile neutropenia
  - In the absence of any obvious source, administration of empiric antibiotic with antipseudomonal activity should be initiated immediately after obtaining blood cultures (peripheral and from indwelling catheter if any).

- Oral antibiotics could be used for low-risk patients (outpatient at the time of developing fever, anticipated to recover from neutropenia within 1 week, good performance status, no associated acute comorbidities such as hepatic/renal insufficiency). A common oral regimen is ciprofloxacin 750 mg PO BID plus amoxicillin/clavulanate 875 mg PO BID.
- Intravenous antibiotics should be used for high-risk patients (inpatient at time of developing fever, significant medical comorbidity or clinically unstable, anticipated prolonged duration of neutropenia ≥7 days, hepatic/renal insufficiency, uncontrolled/progressive cancer). Parenteral antibiotic options include imipenem/cilastatin 500 mg IV q6h, meropenem 1 g IV q8h, piperacillin/tazobactam 4.5 g IV q6h, cefepime 2 g IV q8h, and ceftazidime 2 g IV q8h.
- Vancomycin should be added if central venous access infection is suspected, there is a history of recent methicillin-resistant *Staphylococcus aureus* (MRSA) infection, or the blood culture is positive for Gram-positive cocci.
- Consider antifungal therapy (e.g., voriconazole 6 mg/kg IV q12h) if fever and neutropenia are persistent after 3–5 days of empiric antibacterial therapy.
- Consider antiviral therapy (e.g., acyclovir 10 mg/kg IV q8h) if herpes simplex virus/varicella zoster virus (HSV/VZV) infection is suspected.

Management for Patients with Months of Life Expectancy

- Management is similar to patients with years of life expectancy. Empiric antibiotic therapy is indicated.

Management for Patients with Weeks/Days of Life Expectancy

- At the end of life, antibiotics may still have a role to control life-threatening infections and to improve symptom control. Their use needs to be balanced against the need for hospitalization, diagnostic tests, and potential adverse reactions to antibiotics.

Recommended Reading

1. de Naurois J, et al. Management of febrile neutropenia: ESMO Clinical Practice Guidelines. *Annal Oncol* 2010;21(Suppl 5):v252–256.
2. Nagy-Agren S, et al. Management of infections in palliative care patients with advanced cancer. *J Pain Sympt Manage* 2002;24(1):64–70.

Chapter 29

Thrombocytopenia

Daniel E. Epner

Classification

- Decreased platelet production—Marrow injury by myelosuppressive drugs (such as chemotherapy) or irradiation, aplastic anemia, megaloblastic hematopoiesis (B_{12} or folate deficiency), marrow infiltration by tumor, lymphoma, or leukemia
- Increased platelet destruction—Disseminated intravascular coagulation (DIC), thrombotic thrombocytopenic purpura (TTP), hemolytic-uremic syndrome, platelet damage by abnormal vascular surfaces, infection, autoimmune [idiopathic, secondary (infections, pregnancy, collagen vascular disorders, lymphoproliferative disorders, drugs (heparin, for instance)]
- Abnormal platelet distribution or pooling: Disorders of the spleen (neoplastic, congestive, infiltrative, infectious)
- Artifactual thrombocytopenia: Platelet clumping in the test tube caused by anticoagulant-dependent immunoglobulin (pseudothrombocytopenia)

Symptoms and Signs

- Petechiae
- Superficial ecchymoses
- Persistent bleeding from superficial cuts and scratches
- Persistent or recurrent gastrointestinal bleeding, epistaxis, or hematuria
- Coexistence of bleeding and thromboembolic phenomena or bleeding from previously intact venipuncture sites is suggestive of DIC.

Investigations

- Peripheral blood smear
  - Pseudothrombocytopenia due to *in vitro* platelet clumping when EDTA is used as an anticoagulant. Platelet count will normalize with citrated blood.
  - Schistocytes visible in DIC, TTP—Hemolytic uremic syndrome (HUS)
  - All cell lines are affected by chemotherapy.
- Bone marrow aspiration is usually not necessary if diagnosis is apparent from history, physical examination, laboratory data, and blood smear.

Table 29.1 Thrombocytopenia and Associated Laboratory Findings

Condition	Laboratory Findings
Disseminated intravascular coagulation (DIC)	• Positive DIC panel [elevated prothrombin time/partial thromboplastin time (PT/PTT), D-dimers, fibrin degradation products; low fibrinogen] • Schistocytes on peripheral smear • Possibly evidence of hemolysis [low haptoglobin, positive coombs, high lactate dehydrogenase (LDH), and direct bilirubin]
Chemotherapy-induced thrombocytopenia	• Associated with leukopenia and anemia typically 7–10 days after chemotherapy
Heparin-induced thrombocytopenia (HIT)	• ELISA assay for antiplatelet factor 4-heparin • IgG antibody
Thrombotic thrombocytopenic purpura (TTP)–hemolytic uremic syndrome (HUS)	• Schistocytes on smear, normal coagulation parameters, laboratory values consistent with hemolysis (see DIC above) renal insufficiency
Immune thrombocytopenic purpura (ITP)	• If seen in association with autoimmune hemolytic anemia: Evans syndrome

Distinguishes conditions associated with peripheral platelet consumption [such as DIC, TTP, immune thrombocytopenic purpura (ITP)] from those associated with reduced production (such as chemotherapy-induced thrombocytopenia or marrow infiltration by malignant process or less commonly infection) (Table 29.1).

Relevance to the Cancer Palliative Care Setting

• Thrombocytopenia may occur as a result of intensive cancer treatments such as chemotherapy or radiation or result from marrow infiltration by tumor or infection. Several drugs commonly used in palliative care, such as haloperidol, may also cause thrombocytopenia.

• Thrombocytopenia may complicate the care of cancer patients at the end of life.

  • Anticoagulants and nonsteroidal antiinflammatory drugs (NSAIDs) should be avoided in patients with thrombocytopenia <50,000/μL.

  • Suppositories and enemas are generally contraindicated with severe thrombocytopenia (<10,000/μL).

  • Common procedures such as the placement of permanent or temporary central venous catheters, transbronchial and esophageal endoscopic biopsies, paranasal sinus aspirations, bone marrow biopsies, and occasionally even major surgery may be conducted in patients with advanced cancer. A platelet count of 40,000/μL to 50,000/μL is sufficient to perform major invasive procedures with safety in the absence of associated coagulation abnormalities. Certain procedures, such as bone marrow aspirations and biopsies, can be performed safely at counts of less than 20,000/μL.

Management for Patients with Years of Life Expectancy

- Acute bleeding episode: Transfuse random donor platelet concentrate or single donor platelets produced by apheresis. Single donor platelets are more expensive.
- Prophylactic versus therapeutic platelet transfusion: Prophylactic platelet transfusion should be administered to patients with thrombocytopenia resulting from impaired bone marrow function to reduce the risk of hemorrhage when the platelet count falls below a predefined threshold level. This threshold level for transfusion varies according to the patient's diagnosis, clinical condition, and treatment modality.
    - Acute Leukemia:
    - Threshold of 10,000/μL for prophylactic platelet transfusion in adult patients receiving therapy for acute leukemia.
    - Higher threshold for patients with fever, concurrent coagulopathy, hyperleukocytosis, rapid decline in platelet count, undergoing invasive procedure, or receiving heparin.
- Recipients of high-dose therapy with stem-cell support: Such patients may experience more mucosal injury than patients receiving conventional antileukemic chemotherapy. Nonetheless, guidelines for prophylactic transfusion similar to those for patients with acute leukemia can be used in transplant recipients, with similar caveats about transfusion at higher counts in patients with complicating clinical conditions.
- Patients with chronic, stable, severe thrombocytopenia (for instance, those with myelodysplasia or aplastic anemia): Many such patients have minimal or no significant bleeding for long periods of time despite low platelet counts. Many of these patients can be observed without prophylactic transfusion, reserving platelet transfusions for episodes of hemorrhage or during times of active treatment.
- Patients with solid tumors (chemotherapy-induced thrombocytopenia): Prophylactic transfusion at a threshold of 10,000/μL platelets or less. Consider a threshold of 20,000/μL for patients receiving aggressive therapy for bladder tumors as well as those with demonstrated necrotic tumors, due to their presumed increased risk of bleeding at these sites.
- Patients with alloimmune refractory thrombocytopenia: Transfuse platelets from donors who are HLA-A and HLA-B antigen selected. For patients whose HLA type cannot be determined, or who have uncommon HLA types for which suitable donors cannot be identified, or who do not respond to HLA matched platelets, histocompatible platelet donors can often be identified using platelet cross-matching techniques.

Management for Patients with Months of Life Expectancy

- Management is similar to patients with years of life expectancy.

Management for Patients with Weeks/Days of Life Expectancy

- At the end of life, avoid frequent blood work and other diagnostic tests if possible. Carefully weigh the potential risks and benefits of any intervention. The focus shifts entirely to comfort and dignity.
- Many patients enter home hospice programs and typically forego transfusions, intravenous antibiotics, chemotherapy, radiation, or invasive procedures and opt instead to spend as much time as possible with loved ones at home.

Recommended Reading

1. Schiffer CA, Anderson KC, Bennett CL, et al. Platelet transfusion for patients with cancer: clinical practice guidelines of the American Society of Clinical Oncology. *J Clin Oncol* 2001;19(5):1519–1538.

2. Sekhon SS, Roy V. Thrombocytopenia in adults: a practical approach to evaluation and management. *South Med J* 2006(5);99:491–498.

3. Greer JP, et al. (eds.). *Wintrobe's Clinical Hematology* (12th ed.). Lippincott Williams & Wilkins, Philadelphia, PA, 2009.

Chapter 30

Bleeding Disorders

Marieberta Vidal

Classification

- Localized—Tumor invasion of vessels, tumor surface bleeding
- Systemic—Thrombocytopenia, platelet dysfunction, disseminated intravascular coagulopathy (DIC), coagulation protein defects, concomitant diseases

Symptoms and Signs

- Symptoms—Petechias, bruises, hematomas, menorrhagia, hemarthrosis, hematemesis, hematochezia, melena, hemoptysis, hematuria, epistaxis, excessive bleeding after minor trauma or surgery
- Signs—Tachycardia, hypotension, fever, pain, dyspnea

Investigations

- Laboratory data—Platelet count, bleeding time (BT), prothrombin time (PT), activated partial thromboplastin time (aPTT), and thrombin time (TT), peripheral smear, platelet aggregation, coagulation factor assays, fibrin split products, and D-dimer levels.
- If internal or intracranial bleeding is suspected radiologic investigation is warranted.

Relevance to Cancer Palliative Care Settings

- Hemorrhage occurs in approximately 6–10% of patients with advanced cancer, but the incidence of terminal hemorrhage is approximately 3–12%.
- Visible bleeding can be particularly distressing to patients and their caregivers.

Management for Patients with Years of Life Expectancy

- Local interventions
  - Packing and dressings—Use to achieve hemostasis in vaginal, rectal, and nasal bleeding.

- Hemostatic agents—Epinephrine, prostaglandins, silver nitrate, formalin, aluminum astringents, and sucralfate.
- Radiotherapy—May be useful for hemoptysis, cancerous lesions in the vagina, rectum, and skin, hematuria from bladder cancer, head and neck cancers, and upper gastrointestinal lesions.
- Endoscopy—Banding for variceal bleeding, electrocautery of gastrointestinal, lung, and bladder lesions.
- Interventional radiology—Transcutaneous arterial embolization (TAE), intractable hemorrhage from pelvic urologic malignancies, carotid artery rupture, or spontaneous rupture of hepatocellular carcinoma.
- Surgical interventions—Ligation of major vessels and/or removal of bleeding tissue. Reserved for patients who failed conservative measures and with good performance status.
- Systemic pharmacologic interventions (Table 30.1)
  - Hold anticoagulants and other agents that increase the risk of bleeding.
  - Vasopressin/demopressin—Cause splanchnic arteriolar vasoconstriction, used in variceal bleeding and upper gastrointestinal malignancies.
  - Vitamin K—For prolonged PT, PTT, and INR, reverse excessive warfarin.
  - Somatostatin analogues—Reduce splanchnic flow and pressure.
  - Antifibrinolytic agents—Block the binding sites of plasminogen and decrease lysis.
  - Blood products—Fresh frozen plasma, coagulation factors, pack red blood cells, and platelet transfusion.

Management for Patients with Months of Life Expectancy

- The management of bleeding disorders in patients with months of life expectancy is the same as with years of life expectancy.

Table 30.1 Common Medications for Bleeding Disorders

Drug Class	Drugs and Dosages
Tranexamic acid	1.5 g PO × 1 dose then 1 g PO TID
Aminocaproic acid	Acute bleeding: Loading dose: 4–5 g IV during the first hour, followed by 1 g/h (or 1.25 g/h using oral solution) for 8 h or until bleeding is controlled (maximum daily dose: 30 g)
	Control of bleeding with severe thrombocytopenia
	Initial: 100 mg/kg (maximum 5 g) IV over 30–60 min Maintenance: 1–4 g PO every 4–8 h or 1 g/h IV (maximum daily dose: 24 g)
Vasopressin	0.4 units IV bolus followed by infusion of 0.4 to 1 unit/min
Octreotide	50µg IV bolus followed by 50 µg/h
Vitamin K	10 mg IV × 1 over 1 h for life threatening or serious bleeding
	2.5 mg to 5 mg PO q12–24 h to correct INR without significant bleeding

Management of Patients with Weeks/Days of Life Expectancy

- The issue of aggressive procedures and ongoing transfusions at the end of life poses an ethical dilemma because survival may not be prolonged if the cause of bleeding (i.e., cancer) cannot be easily reversed. Sensitive and emphatic discussions with patients and families and physicians are essential.
- If using a palliative approach, the focus should be on controlling the bleeding without resuscitative measures.
- In patients with high risk of major bleeding complications, healthcare professionals and caregivers need to be prepared.
  - Use dark towels to absorb blood and apply pressure.
  - If major hematemesis or hemoptysis occurs, place the patient in a lateral position on the side of the bleed.
  - If intractable bleeding is a major source of distress or discomfort for the patient, sedatives such as benzodiazepines are indicated.

Recommended Reading

1. Pereira J, Phan T. Management of bleeding in patients with advanced cancer. *Oncologist* 2004;9(5):561–570.

2. Pereira J, Mancini I, Bruera E. The management of bleeding in patients with advanced cancer. In Portenoy RK, Bruera E (eds.). *Topics in Palliative Care* (Vol. 4). Oxford University Press, New York, 2000: 163–183.

3. Gagnon B, Mancini I, Pereira J, et al. Palliative management of bleeding events in advanced cancer patients. *J Palliat Care* 1998;14:50–54.

4. Harris DG, Noble SIR. Management of terminal hemorrhage in patients with advanced cancer: a systematic review. *J Pain Sympt Manage* 2009;38(6): 913–927.

Chapter 31

Deep Venous Thrombosis

Marieberta Vidal

Classification

Deep venous thrombosis (DVT) is the formation of a thrombus in a deep vein, predominantly in the legs, although it can also occur in the upper extremities.

- Upper extremities DVT: Are approximately 10% of the cases, more common now with the use of central venous catheters.
- Lower extremity DVT:
  - Distal (below the knee)—The thrombi remain in the deep calf veins.
  - Proximal (above the knee)—Involves the iliac, femoral, and popliteal veins.
- Acute DVT: The symptoms appear around 5–7 days after the event and are usually occlusive and more symptomatic.
- Chronic DVT: Symptomatic DVT that persists for longer than 10–14 days is usually nonocclusive.

Symptoms and Signs

- Symptoms—Pain and swelling of the extremity
- Signs—Edema, warmth, erythema, and/or superficial vein dilatation

Investigations

- Doppler ultrasonography is the most common noninvasive test used for the diagnosis of DVT.
- If a noninvasive test is not conclusive, venography may be used.
- D-dimer assays are helpful for screening but are not diagnostics. D-dimer is usually elevated at levels greater than 500 ng/mL of fibrinogen equivalent units in nearly all patients with venous thromboembolism. However, it can be elevated just due to malignancy, recent surgery, and other comorbidities.

Relevance to Cancer Palliative Care Settings

- Patients with advanced cancer are at high risk for DVT due to the hypercoagulable state from the malignancy itself. This risk increased even more with the use of certain antineoplastic treatments, catheters, surgeries, infections, and immobilization.

- DVT may affect the patient's quality of life as it might cause pain and swelling and decrease mobility. If the clot migrates and the patient develops a pulmonary embolism not only could the symptom burden increase but it can also cause death.

Management for Patients with Years of Life Expectancy

- The treatment of DVT is indicated mainly to prevent or treat complications such as pulmonary embolism, extension of the clot, recurrent thromboembolic events, and improvement of current symptoms.
- Common treatments are listed in Tables 31.1 and 31.2. Novel oral anticoagulants such as rivaroxaban, dabigatran, and apixaban can be given in fixed doses without monitoring. However, there is inadequate evidence to support their use for prevention or treatment of venous thromboembolism in the palliative care setting.
- Duration of anticoagulation:
  - For the first episode of DVT in the general population, anticoagulation for 3 months is recommended.
  - Because the risk of recurrent venous thromboembolism is very high in patients with active cancer, it is recommended that they receive anticoagulation for over 3 months if the risk of bleeding is not high.
  - For patients with advanced metastatic cancer, indefinite anticoagulation is suggested unless they develop bleeding complications or request discontinuation for quality of life reasons.
- Absolute contraindications for anticoagulation include intracranial bleeding, severe active bleeding, recent brain, eye, or spinal cord surgery, pregnancy, and malignant hypertension. Relative contraindications include recent major surgery, a recent cerebrovascular accident, and severe thrombocytopenia. The platelet count threshold for anticoagulation has not been established in the literature. However, the risk of bleeding increases significantly when the platelet count drops below 50,000.

Table 31.1 Short-Term Pharmacologic Anticoagulation

Agent	Common Doses
Dalteparin	200 units/kg subcutaneous daily
Enoxaparin	1 mg/kg subcutaneous daily
Tinzaparin	175 units/kg subcutaneous daily
Fondaparinux	5 mg (<50 kg), 7.5 mg (50–100 kg), 10 mg (>100 kg) subcutaneous daily
Unfractionated heparin	80 units/kg load IV, then 18 units/kg/h to target a partial thromboplastin time (PTT) of 2–2.5 × control

Table 31.2 Long-Term Pharmacologic Anticoagulation

Agent	Common Doses
Low-molecular-weight heparin	Proximal or recurrent deep venous thrombosis (DVT)
	Preferred for the first 6 months
Warfarin	Initiated with an agent of the acute treatment
	Target INR between 2 and 3

- Inferior vena cava (IVC) filters may be considered in patients who have lower extremity DVT and an absolute contraindication to anticoagulation (e.g., active bleeding, recent surgery, hemorrhagic stroke). Upon resolution of the contraindication, anticoagulation is recommended despite placement of the IVC.
- For upper extremity DVT, the treatment goal is to relieve acute symptoms and to prevent embolization. Anticoagulation is recommended for DVT of axillary or more proximal veins. The catheter can be left in place if functional and necessary.

Management for Patients with Months of Life Expectancy

- The management plan is similar to that of patients with years of life expectancy. Anticoagulation is indicated unless the patient has contraindications.

Management of Patients with Weeks/Days of Life Expectancy

- At the end of life the treatment of DVT needs to be individualized. The main objective is to decrease symptom burden and to improve quality of life. In this context the decision will depend on professional experience, patient's preferences, plan of care, performance status, and severity of symptoms caused by the DVT.
- The need for anticoagulation needs to be constantly reevaluated due to the rapid evolving clinical scenario in these patients.
- Patients near the end of life might not be able to swallow pills. They can develop renal insufficiency that limits the use of low-molecular-weight heparin.

Recommended Reading

1. Noble SI, Shelley MD, Coles B, et al. Management of venous thromboembolism in patients with advanced cancer: a systematic review and meta-analysis. *Lancet Oncol* 2008;9:577.

2. Streiff MB, Chair. Venous thromboembolic disease, version 2.2011. National Comprehensive Cancer Network (NCCN) guidelines are available online at www.nccn.org.

3. Djulbegovic B. Management of venous thromboembolism in cancer: a brief review of risk-benefit approaches and guidelines' recommendations. *J Support Oncol* 2010;8:84.

4. Farge D, Debourdeau P, Beckers M, et al. International clinical practice guidelines for the treatment and prophylaxis of venous thromboembolism in patients with cancer. *J Thromb Haemost* 2013;11:56.

Section VII

Infections

Chapter 32

Sepsis

Susan Gaeta

Classification

- Systemic inflammatory response syndrome (SIRS)—Two or more of the following:
  - Heart rate greater than or equal to 90 beats/min
  - Temperature greater than 38°C or less than 36°C
  - Respiratory rate greater than or equal to 20 breaths/min
  - White blood cell (WBC) greater than or equal to 12,000/mL or less than or equal to 4,000/mL
- Sepsis—Systemic inflammatory response syndrome (SIRS) due to a documented or presumed infection
- Severe sepsis—Sepsis-induced tissue hypoperfusion or organ dysfunction
- Septic shock—Sepsis with hypotension that is refractory despite adequate fluid resuscitation

Symptoms and Signs

- Symptoms—Nonspecific but may include confusion, delirium, weakness, nausea, vomiting, abdominal pain, cough
- Signs—Tachycardia, hyperthermia, hypothermia, tachypnea, cold extremities, oliguria, anuria, hypotension, skin mottling, hypoxemia

Investigations

- Lactic acid, complete blood count (CBC), arterial blood gas, serum chemistry panel, prothrombin time (PT), partial thromboplastin time (PTT), international normalized ratio (INR), fibrinogen.
- Obtain cultures from blood, urine, sputum, and other sources but a delay in the administration of appropriate antibiotics for more than an hour can result in an increase in mortality.
- Radiologic imaging as needed to identify the source of infection.

Relevance to the Cancer Palliative Care Setting

• Cancer patients are 10 times more likely to develop sepsis then noncancer patients because of their immunosuppressed state due to chemotherapy and/or underlying malignancy.

• Since the signs and symptoms of sepsis are nonspecific, it is important to consider sepsis in the differential diagnosis of patients with acute deterioration.

• Early diagnosis and treatment of sepsis are essential to reducing the risk of progression to severe sepsis and/or septic shock, which in turn would lower the need for an intensive care unit admission and decrease mortality from sepsis.

• The case-fatality rate from sepsis in cancer patients has been reported to be 55% higher than noncancer patients.

Management for Patients with Years of Life Expectancy

• The mortality rate in patients presenting with sepsis is 41% at 1 month, 65% at 6 months, and 72% at 1 year. For cancer patients who otherwise are expected to have a reasonable life expectancy, management should be identical to that for patients without cancer.

• Broad-spectrum antibiotics: The exact treatment varies depending on local resistance patterns and drug availability.

• Identify and remove the source of infection if possible, i.e., drainage of abscess, surgical intervention, removal of indwelling catheters.

• Intravenous fluid challenge of 30 mL/kg over 30–60 minutes, may repeat if the mean arterial pressure (MAP) is less than 65. Monitor SpO_2 during fluid challenge.

• Vasopressor support with norepinephrine if the MAP is less than 65 despite fluid resuscitation.

• The patient may need to be transferred to the ICU for vasopressor support, respiratory support, and/or invasive hemodynamic monitoring.

• Discuss goals of care and prognosis within 72 hours of admission.

Management for Patients with Months of Life Expectancy

• Management is similar to patients with years of life expectancy.

• Discussion of care goals and advance care planning should have taken place while the patients were well. By the time sepsis occurs, it may sometimes be too late to have an in-depth discussion with the patient about goals of care. If patients are too ill to participate in decision making, surrogate decision makers should be involved.

• Discussions should include how aggressive patients should be managed if they progressed from sepsis to severe sepsis to septic shock. In particular, the risks and benefits of invasive monitoring and/or endotracheal intubation need to be addressed.

Management for Patients with Weeks/Days of Life Expectancy

- For patients with rapidly progressive cancer despite multiple lines of prior therapies, poor baseline performance status, and a life expectancy in weeks or less who subsequently develop sepsis, aggressive measures such as intensive care unit admissions, mechanical ventilation, and invasive monitoring may not be warranted because of the low benefit-to-risk ratio. Even if sepsis can be treated, the advanced cancer is usually resistant and often not reversible.
- It would be imperative to have goals of care and code status discussions long before the occurrence of sepsis in these individuals and to have continual dialogue with patients and their families throughout the hospital admission. If comfort care is chosen, it may still be possible to continue antibiotics and other symptom support measures while keeping patients in the acute care units, palliative care units, or even at home.

Recommended Reading

1. Danai PA, Moss M, et al. The epidemiology of sepsis in patients with malignancy. *Chest* 2006;129(6):1432–1440.

2. Dellinger RP, Levy M, et al. Surviving Sepsis Campaign: international Guidelines for Management of Severe Sepsis and Septic Shock: 2012. *CCM* 2012;41(2):580–637.

Chapter 33

Pneumonia

Shalini Dalal

Classification

- Community-acquired pneumonia (CAP)—Bacterial pathogens are the most common cause and include "typical" (*Streptococcus pneumoniae, Haemophilus influenzae, Staphylococcus aureus*, Group A streptococci, *Moraxella catarrhalis*, anaerobes, and aerobic Gram-negative bacteria) and "atypical" pathogens (*Legionella* spp., *Mycoplasma pneumoniae, Chlamydophila pneumoniae*, and *Chlamydophila psittaci*). *Staphylococcus pneumoniae* is the most common cause of CAP.
- Nosocomial or hospital-acquired pneumonia (HAP)—Acquired 48 hours or more after admission and did not appear to be incubating at the time of admission. It is the leading cause of death among hospital-acquired infections. It is classified as early-onset (within 96 hours) or late-onset (>96 hours after admission) and is latter associated with higher multidrug-resistant (MDR) pathogens, morbidity, and mortality.
- Ventilator-associated pneumonia (VAP)—It is a subset of HAP; it develops > 48 hours after endotracheal intubation.
- Healthcare-associated pneumonia (HCAP)—Occurs in nonhospitalized patients with extensive healthcare contact. Risk factors include hospitalization for ≥2 days within 90 days; resident of long-term care facility; received chemotherapy, intravenous antibiotics, wound care, or dialysis within 30 days; immunosuppressive disease and/or therapy; and family member with MDR pathogen (Box 33.1).

Box 33.1 Risk Factors for Multidrug-Resistant Pathogens Causing Nosocomial Pneumonia

- Current hospitalization of ≥5 days
- High frequency of antibiotic resistance in the community/specific hospital unit
- Presence of risk factors for healthcare-acquired pneumonia (HCAP) (see text), includes cancer patients with recent/undergoing cancer therapy

---

Symptoms and Signs

- Fever, chills, cough, purulent sputum, dyspnea, and pleuritic chest pain.
- Older patients may not exhibit the above, and often present with weakness, decline in functional status, and altered mentation.
- Physical examination may reveal tachycardia, tachypnea, chest dullness to percussion, egophony, rales, or bronchial breaths sounds.

Investigations

- Comprehensive medical history and physical examination to evaluate infection severity, exclude other sources of infection, and review of comorbidities that may influence etiologic pathogens.
- Chest radiograph: Posteroanterior and lateral views are preferable unless intubated. May demonstrate the presence/severity of unilobar or multilobar infiltrates or consolidation as well as complications such as cavitation or effusions.
- Arterial oxygenation to determine the need for supplemental oxygen.
- Arterial blood gasses (ABGs) if metabolic or respiratory acidosis is suspected and for intensive care unit (ICU) patients.
- Sputum cultures: Recommended prior to antibiotic administration in all patients with hospital-acquired pneumonia (HAP) and hypoplastic coronary artery disease (HCAD) and selected hospitalized patients with community-acquired pneumonia (CAP) (ICU admission, failed outpatient antibiotics, cavitary lesion or pleural effusion on imaging, severe underlying lung disease, active alcohol abuse).
- Urine antigen testing for *Pneumococcus* and *Legionella* for CAP (ICU admission, failed outpatient antibiotics, pleural effusion on imaging, severe underlying lung disease, active alcohol abuse). In addition, asplenic patients should have *Pneumococcus* testing.
- CBC, electrolytes, and renal and liver function to rule out multiorgan dysfunction in patients meeting the criteria for admission.

Relevance to the Cancer Palliative Care Setting

- Pneumonia occurs frequently in cancer patients with advanced illness due to their immunosuppressed state and frequent need for hospitalizations. It is also a frequent cause of death in cancer patients.
- Neutropenic cancer patients are more susceptible to infection with resistant pathogens and are at increased risk for septicemia.

Management of Patients with Years of Life Expectancy

- Hospitalization is recommended for high-risk patients with HCAP or HAP when MDR pathogens are suspected or when patients are neutropenic (see Chapter 28). In patients with CAP, prognostic models such as the Pneumonia

Table 33.1 Initial Empiric Antibiotic Therapy for Community Acquired Pneumonia

Classification	Empiric Antibiotic Selection
Outpatient healthy no antibiotic use in 90 days	Macrolide (azithromycin) *or* Doxycycline
Outpatient Comorbidities (diabetes, malignancy, chronic heart, lung, liver, or renal disease immunosuppressing conditions or therapies antibiotic use in 90 days	Respiratory fluoroquinolone (moxifloxacin, levofloxacin) *or* β-Lactam (amoxicillin/clavulanate) plus macrolide (azithromycin)
Inpatient, non-intensive care unit (ICU)	Respiratory fluoroquinolone (moxifloxacin, levofloxacin) *or* β-Lactam (ceftriaxone, cefotaxime, or ampicillin/sulbactam) plus macrolide (azithromycin) If methicillin-resistant *Staphylococcus aureas* (MRSA) is suspected add vancomycin or linezolid
Inpatient ICU	β-Lactam antibiotic (ceftriaxone, cefotaxime, or ampicillin/sulbactam) *plus* Azithromycin or a respiratory fluoroquinolone (moxifloxacin, levofloxacin) If MRSA is suspected add vancomycin or linezolid

Severity Index (PSI) can be used to identify patients for inpatient management (PSI > 2). In addition, patients with compliance concerns or inadequate social support should be admitted.

• Empiric antibiotic regimens are shown in Tables 33.1 and 33.2.

Management for Patients with Months of Life Expectancy

• The general approach is similar to that of patients with years to live.

Management for Patients with Weeks/Days of Life Expectancy

• At the end of life the focus shifts to control of distressful symptoms. Clinicians should elicit patient preferences for treatment of infections and discuss symptom control as the major indication for antibiotic use. Although limited, most studies conducted in terminally ill cancer patients receiving hospice care suggest that antibiotic treatment of respiratory tract infections has variable success

Table 33.2 Initial Empiric Antibiotic Therapy for Hospital-Acquired Pneumonia, Ventilator-Associated Pneumonia, and Healthcare-Associated Pneumonia

Classification	Potential Pathogens	Empiric Antibiotic Selection
Early onset and no risk of multidrug-resistant (MDR) pathogens	Streptococcus pneumoniae Haemophilus influenzae Methicillin-sensitive Staphylococcus aureus Antibiotic-sensitive enteric Gram-negative bacilli (Escherichia coli, Klebsiella pneumoniae, Enterobacter species, Proteus species, Serratia marcescens)	Ceftriaxone or fluoroquinolones (levofloxacin, moxifloxacin, ciprofloxacin) or ampicillin/sulbactam or ertapenem
Late onset or risk of MDR pathogens	As above and Pseudomonas aeruginosa Klebsiella pneumoniae Acinetobacter species Methicillin-resistant Staphylococcus aureus (MRSA)	Antipseudomonal cephalosporin (cefepime, ceftazidime) or Antipseudomonal carbepenem (imipenem or meropenem) or β-Lactam/β-lactamase inhibitor (piperacillin–tazobactam) Plus either Antipseudomonal fluoroquinolone (ciprofloxacin or levofloxacin) or Aminoglycoside (amikacin, gentamicin, or tobramycin) Plus Linezolid or vancomycin

in symptom control and survival. With or without antibiotics, symptom control measures should be offered to patients for cough, fever, dyspnea, or pain.

Recommended Reading

1. Niederman MS, Craven DE, Bonten MJ, et al. American Thoracic Society and the Infectious Diseases Society of America Guidelines for the management of adults with hospital-acquired, ventilator-associated, and healthcare-associated pneumonia. Am J Respir Crit Care Med 2005;171:388–416.

2. Mandell LA, Wunderink RG, Anzueto A, et al. Infectious Diseases Society of America/American Thoracic Society consensus guidelines on the management of community-acquired pneumonia in adults. Clin Infect Dis 2007;44(Suppl 2):S27–S72.

3. Reinbolt RE, Shenk AM, White PH, Navari RM. Symptomatic treatment of infections in patients with advanced cancer receiving hospice care. J Pain Symptom Manage 2005;30:175–182.

Chapter 34

Urinary Tract Infections

Shalini Dalal

Classification

- Urinary tract infections (UTIs) include infections localized to the lower (cystitis) or upper (pyelonephritis) tract. Both may coexist.
- Uncomplicated, community-acquired UTIs: Most often (80%) these are caused by *Escherichia coli*. Other pathogens include other species of Enterobacteriaceae, such as *Proteus mirabilis, Klebsiella pneumoniae*, and *Staphylococcus saprophyticus*.
- Complicated UTI: These are associated with underlying factors that increase the risk of failing therapy (Box 34.1). Uropathogens are comprised of Gram-negative species in 60–80% (*Escherichia coli*, followed by *Klebsiella, Pseudomonas, Proteus*, and *Enterobacter*) and Gram-positive pathogens in 20–40% (enterococci and staphylococci) of instances and are inherently more resistant to antibiotics.

157

Symptoms and Signs

- Cystitis: Dysuria, frequency, urgency, suprapubic pain, and/or hematuria.
- Pyelonephritis: Symptoms of cystitis such as fever (>38°C), chills, flank pain, costovertebral angle tenderness/pain, and nausea/vomiting may or may not be present.
- Symptoms can be subtle in the very young and very old.

Investigations

- Urine culture and a susceptibility test should be performed in patients with complicating features (Box 34.1), risk for antibiotic resistance, and when pyelonephritis is suspected prior to empiric antibiotic administration.

Box 34.1 Factors Associated with Complicated Urinary Tract Infections

- Nosocomial acquired urinary tract infections
- Structural abnormalities such as calculi, tract anomalies, indwelling catheter, stent, nephrostomy tube, and urinary tract obstruction
- Metabolic disease such as diabetes and renal insufficiency; pregnancy
- Impaired host defenses such as HIV, current chemotherapy, underlying active cancer

- Urine analysis (by microscopy or dipstick) may be sufficient for the diagnosis of uncomplicated cystitis if symptoms are consistent with UTI.
- Radiographic imaging: Computed tomography (CT) scan is preferred to detect complicated UTI. It should be considered in patients with persistent symptoms after 2–3 days of appropriate antibiotic treatment for acute uncomplicated UTI and in patients with pyelonephritis to rule out complicated pyelonephritis.

Relevance to the Cancer Palliative Care Setting

- UTIs occur frequently and are more severe in oncology and palliative care patients due to compromised immune systems and the frequent need for hospitalizations and indwelling urinary catheters.

Table 34.1 Empiric Antibiotic Regimen

Urinary Tract Infection	Empiric Antibiotic Selection
Uncomplicated acute bacterial cystitis	Treatment in women 3 days, men 7 days
	Trimethoprim/sulfamethoxazole 160 mg/800 mg PO BID
	If resistance (>15–20%) to above, consider one of the following:
	Ciprofloxacin 250 mg PO BID or norfloxacin 400 mg PO BID or ofloxacin 200 mg PO BID or levofloxacin 250 mg PO daily or augmentin 875 mg PO BID or 500 mg PO TID
Complicated cystitis	Fluoroquinolones are the preferred agents:
	Ciprofloxacin 500 mg PO BID ×7 d or levofloxacin 750 mg PO daily ×5 d
	In hospitalized patients: IV may be switched to PO when appropriate, total of 7–14 d Levofloxacin 500 mg IV daily or ceftriaxone 1 g IV daily or meropenem 500 mg IV q8h OR an aminoglycoside (3–5 mg/kg of gentamicin or tobramycin)
Uncomplicated pyelonephritis	Fluoroquinolones are the preferred agents:
	Ciprofloxacin 500 mg PO BID ×7 d or levofloxacin 750 mg PO daily ×5 d
	If fluoroquinolone resistance >10%:
	A single dose of 1 g IV ceftriaxone or a consolidated 24 h dose of an aminoglycoside (gentamicin 7 mg/kg IV or tobramycin 7 mg/kg IV or amikacin 20 mg/kg IV) and trimethoprim/sulfamethoxazole (160 mg/800 mg) 1 tablet PO BID for 14 d
Complicated pyelonephritis	Mild to moderate illness (one of the following):
	Ceftriaxone 1 g IV q24h or cefepime 1 g IV q12h or ciprofloxacin 400 mg IV q12 h or levofloxacin 750 mg IV q24 h or aztreonam 1 g IV q8 to 12h
	Severe illness immunocompromise and/or incomplete urinary drainage (one of the following):
	Ampicillin-sulbactam 1.5 g IV q6h or ticarcillin-clavulanate 3.1 g IV q6h or piperacillin-tazobactam 3.375 g IV q6h or meropenem 500 mg IV q8h or imipenem 500 mg IV q6h or doripenem 500 mg IV q8h

- Neutropenic cancer patients are more susceptible to infections with resistant pathogens. UTIs may not manifest with dysuria or pyuria in neutropenic patients, and patients are at increased risk of septicemia.

Management of Patients with Years of Life Expectancy

- For the management of patients with years of life expectancy see Table 34.1.

Management for Patients with Months of Life Expectancy

- The general approach is similar to that for patients with years to live.

Management for Patients with Weeks/Days of Life Expectancy

- At the end of life, the focus shifts to control of distressful symptoms. Hospice clinicians should illicit patient preferences for treatment of infections.
- Although few studies are available in this population, the existing literature suggests that antibiotic treatment for UTIs can improve symptoms in a majority of patients. Given the favorable risk–benefit ratio, empiric antibiotics along with other symptom control measures should be offered to symptomatic patients with UTI.

Recommended Reading

1. Wagenlehner FM, Naber KG: Antibiotic treatment for urinary tract infections: pharmacokinetic/pharmacodynamic principles. *Expert Rev Anti Infect Ther* 2004;2:923–231.

2. Gupta K, Hooton TM, Naber KG, et al: International clinical practice guidelines for the treatment of acute uncomplicated cystitis and pyelonephritis in women: A 2010 update by the Infectious Diseases Society of America and the European Society for Microbiology and Infectious Diseases. *Clin Infect Dis* 2011;52:e103–120.

3. Hooton TM, Bradley SF, Cardenas DD, et al. Diagnosis, prevention, and treatment of catheter-associated urinary tract infection in adults: 2009 International Clinical Practice Guidelines from the Infectious Diseases Society of America. *Clin Infect Dis* 2010;50:625–663.

4. Kawashima A, LeRoy AJ. Radiologic evaluation of patients with renal infections. *Infect Dis Clin North Am* 2003;17:433.

5. Reinbolt RE, Shenk AM, White PH, Navari RM. Symptomatic treatment of infections in patients with advanced cancer receiving hospice care. *J Pain Sympt Manage* 2005;30:175–182.

Chapter 35

Osteomyelitis

Joseph Arthur

Classification

- Contiguous spread—Usually polymicrobial. The source may be either out-side the body (e.g., soft-tissue trauma, open fracture, surgery) or from an adjacent focus (soft-tissue infection, dental abscess, decubitus ulcer).
- Hematogenous spread—Usually monomicrobial. Predominantly encoun-tered in the pediatric population.
- Can also be classified as:
  - Acute (less than 2 weeks)
  - Subacute (2–6 weeks)
  - Chronic (more than 6 weeks)
- See Table 35.1 for a list of common organisms implicated in osteomyelitis

Symptoms and Signs

- Local findings (tenderness, warmth, erythema and swelling, draining sinus tract, especially in chronic disease)
- Systemic or constitutional symptoms (fever, rigors)

Table 35.1 Commonly Isolated Microorganisms in Osteomyelitis	
Microorganism	**Associated Features**
Staphylococcus aureus	Most common organism in osteomyelitis
Coagulase-negative Staphylococcus aureus	Foreign body-associated infections
Pseudomonas aeruginosa	Intravenous (IV) drug users and nosocomial infections
Salmonella or streptococcal pneumonia	Sickle cell disease
Bartonella henselae	HIV patients
Pasteurella multocida or Eikenella corrodens	Human or animal bites
Anaerobes	Bites, diabetic foot infections, decubitus infections
Fungal pathogens	Chronically ill patients Patients receiving long-term IV antibiotics Immunocompromised patients

Investigations

- Clinical diagnosis: Positive probe-to-bone test is sufficient for the diagnosis of osteomyelitis.
- If a diabetic foot ulcer is larger than 2 × 2 cm or the bone is palpable, osteomyelitis is likely and additional noninvasive evaluation may not be needed.
- Laboratory data: Markers of an inflammatory response such as leukocytosis; elevated erythrocyte sedimentation rate (ESR) and C-reactive protein (CRP) are nonspecific. Blood cultures are positive in 50% of patients, especially in hematogenous spread and vertebral osteomyelitis.
- Radiograph
  - Magnetic resonance imaging (MRI) is the test of choice and is very sensitive.
  - A computed tomography (CT) scan can be done if MRI is unavailable.
  - Nuclear study (bone scan, gallium scan, and tagged white blood cell scan)
    - This is recommended if MRI is not possible due to metallic stents or other hardware and CT scan is unreliable due to imaging artifacts.
    - More reliable for evaluation of acute infection than chronic infection given its sensitivity for detecting evidence of inflammation.
    - False-positive results may occur with recent trauma or surgery, recently healed osteomyelitis, septic arthritis, degenerative joint disease, bone tumors, Paget disease, and other noninfectious inflammatory bone conditions.
    - False-negative results are seen in areas of relative ischemia.
- Plain x-ray: This is usually normal in early disease; it is mainly useful after 2–6 weeks and therefore is more useful in chronic osteomyelitis.
- Bone biopsy provides a definite diagnosis if an organism is isolated.

Relevance to the Cancer Palliative Care Setting

- Recalcitrant infection that does not respond to conventional therapy should prompt biopsy to evaluate for malignancy.
- Patients with advanced cancer are at risk for osteomyelitis because of immunosuppression (e.g., chemotherapy) and instrumentation.
- Sinus tract formation may be associated with neoplasms, especially in the setting of longstanding infections, and may result in osteomyelitis.
- Squamous cell carcinoma is the most common tumor associated with chronic osteomyelitis. Other tumors include fibrosarcoma, myeloma, lymphoma, plasmacytoma, angiosarcoma, rhabdomyosarcoma, and malignant fibrous histiocytoma.

Management for Patients with Years of Life Expectancy

- Treatment is mainly with prolonged antibiotic therapy and/or aggressive surgical intervention (Table 35.2).

Table 35.2 Suggested Antibiotic Regimens for Commonly Isolated Microorganisms in Osteomyelitis

Microorganism	Suggested Antibiotic Treatment
Staphylococcus aureus or coagulase-negative Staphylococcus (methicillin sensitive)	Naficillin or oxacillin (2 g IV every 6 h) or cefazolin (1–2 g IV every 8 h)
S. aureus or coagulase-negative Staphylococcus (methicillin resistant)	Vancomycin (1 g IV every 12 h)
Streptococcal species	Penicillin G (5 million units IV every 6 h)
Enterobacteriaceae, quinolone susceptible	Fluoroquinolone (ciprofloxacin 750 mg every 12 h)
Enterobacteriaceae, quinolone resistant	Carbapenem (imipenem 500 mg every 6 h)
Pseudomonas aeruginosa	Cefepime or ceftazidine (2 g IV every 8 h ± an aminoglycoside) or Piperacillin-tazobactam (4.5 g IV every 6 h ± an aminoglycoside)
Anaerobes	Clindamycin (600 mg IV every 6–8 h) or Penicillin G (5 million units IV every 6 h)

- The optimal duration of antibiotic therapy is not certain. Usually parenteral antimicrobial therapy is given for at least 6 weeks from the last debridement and 8 weeks or more in vertebral osteomyelitis. Shorter courses may be used after complete surgical debridement or resection of all infected bone.
- Initial treatment with oral antibiotics is usually avoided although fluoroquinolones may sometimes be used for Gram-negative coverage.
- Surgery is usually considered in the following cases: Acute osteomyelitis that fails medical therapy, chronic osteomyelitis, infected prosthesis, complications of pyogenic vertebral osteomyelitis (e.g., epidural abscess, cord compression).
- Adjunctive therapies for osteomyelitis include hyperbaric oxygen and negative pressure wound therapy (vacuum-assisted closure).

Management for Patients with Months of Life Expectancy

- Management is largely the same as for patients with a longer life expectancy.
- However, patients will need ongoing clinical assessments to reevaluate the therapeutic benefit in the context of the patient's overall prognosis coupled with the existing comorbidities and the prevailing circumstances.
  - For example, surgical interventions such as prosthesis for long-term ambulatory function may need to be reconsidered.
  - Investigations aimed at confirming a suspected diagnosis without altering clinical management should be avoided.

Management for Patients with Weeks/Days of Life Expectancy

- Ongoing therapy such as long-term antibiotics and surgery may be unnecessary in most patients with shortened life expectancy, especially once care goals are redefined.
- Efforts should be made to explain the rationale behind discontinuing some long-term medications to prevent the psychological distress usually associated with it.
- Emphasis should rather be placed on interventions aimed at achieving short-term benefits such as management of disease-related odor, pain control, comfortable positioning of the affected limb, and wound care therapy.
- Consider discontinuing frequent blood draws if possible.
- Caregivers should receive basic training and assistance with wound management and other care needs.

Recommended Reading

1. Lew DP, Waldvogel FA. Osteomyelitis current concepts. *N Engl J Med* 1997;336:999–1007.
2. Mader JT, Shirtliff M, Calhoun JH. Staging and staging application in osteomyelitis. *Clin Infect Dis* 1997;25:1303.
3. Lew DP, Waldvogel FA. Osteomyelitis. *N Engl J Med* 1997;336:999.
4. Stevenson J, et al. Managing comorbidities in patients at the end of life. BMJ 2004;329(7471):909–912.
5. Zimmerli W. Vertebral osteomyelitis. *N Engl J Med* 2010;362:1022–1029.

Chapter 36

Skin Infections

Pedro Pérez-Cruz and M. Cristina Ajenjo

Classification

- Skin bacterial infections
  - Primary
    - Cellulitis—Infection of the dermal and subcutaneous layers of skin
    - Erysipela—Infection of the upper dermis with extension into the superficial cutaneous lymphatics caused by group A streptococci
    - Impetigo—Gram-positive bacterial infection of the superficial layers of the epidermis
    - Ecthyma—Ulcerative pyoderma of the skin often caused by group A streptococci
    - Folliculitis—Infection of hair follicles
    - Furunculosis—Isolated abscesses involving hair follicles
    - Carbuncles—Interconnected abscesses of hair follicles
  - Secondary: Diabetic foot, pressure ulcers
  - Necrotizing fasciitis—Infection of the deeper subcutaneous tissues and fascia characterized by extensive and rapidly spreading necrosis and by gangrene of the skin and underlying structures
- Fungal infections—Tinea corporis, tinea cruris, tinea pedis, cutaneous candidiasis
- Viral infections—Orolabial and genital herpes simplex infections, varicella (chickenpox), herpes zoster (shingles)
- Cellulitis and erysipela are the most frequent skin infection in patients with solid tumors. Therefore, this chapter will focus on these infections. Specific microorganisms and initial recommended treatments are described in Table 36.1.

165

Symptoms and Signs of Cellulitis

- Symptoms—Variable depending on the magnitude of local and systemic compromise. Local pain, swelling, redness, and itching are common. Fever, chills, fatigue, and anorexia suggest systemic compromise.
- Signs—Variable depending on the magnitude of local and systemic involvement. Erythema, heat, pustules, necrotic areas, and ulcers may be seen. Fever and hypotension suggest systemic toxicity.

Table 36.1 Skin Infections, Microorganisms, and Treatment

Diagnosis	Common Microorganisms	Recommended First Line Treatment
Cellulitis	MSSA, MRSA, or CA-MRSA *Streptococcus pyogenes*	Systemic penicillin G or oxacillin or first generation cephalosporin. If MRSA or CA-MRSA is suspected consider TMP-SMX, clindamycin, or doxycylin. In severe cases consider vancomycin
Erysipela	MSSA, MRSA, or CA-MRSA *Streptococcus pyogenes*	Systemic penicillin G or oxacillin or first generation cephalosporin. If MRSA or CA-MRSA is suspected, follow the recommendation above
Impetigo and ecthyma	MSSA *Streptococcus pyogenes*	Topical mupirocin 2%
Folliculitis	MSSA *Candida albicans*	Topical mupirocin 2%. Topical antifungals if *C. albicans* is suspected
Furunculosis and carbuncles	MSSA, MRSA, or CA-MRSA	Surgical drainage + systemic oxacillin or first generation cephalosporin. If MRSA or CA-MRSA is suspected, follow the recommendation above
Diabetic foot, with no risk of amputation	MSSA or *Streptococcus*; less often, Gram-negative bacteria or anaerobes	First generation cephalosporin or β-lactamic plus β-lactamase inhibitor or moxifloxacin
Diabetic foot, with risk of amputation	Polymicrobial: MSSA, *S. agalactiae, Enterococcus* sp., Gram negative, and anaerobes	Surgical assessment + glycemic control + IV antibiotics (ampicillin-sulbactam *or* moxifloxacin or clindamicyn + ciprofloxacin *or* carbapenem + vancomycin)
Pressure ulcers	Polymicrobial: Enterobacteria, *Pseudomonas* spp., *Enterococcus* spp., anaerobes	Surgical assessment + wound management + wide spectrum antibiotics. Gram stain and tissue culture required for antibiotic selection
Necrotizing fasciitis	Type I: *Streptococcus* non-A, anaerobes, Enterobacteriae Type II: *Streptococcus* A ± MSSA, MRSA, CA-MRSA	Surgery + IV antibiotics (penicillin + clindamycin + third generation cephalosporin or vancomycin) + ICU admission
Tinea corporis, tinea cruris, tinea pedis	*Trychophyton rubrum, Trychophyton mentagrophytes, Epidermophyton floccosum*	Drying powder and topical antifungals: terbinafine, miconazole, clotrimazole
Cutaneous candidiasis	*Candida albicans*	Topical tx: clotrimazole 1% cream, myconazole 2% cream, or systemic tx: fluconazole once a week dose, 2 doses
Orolabial or genital herpes	Herpes simplex virus 1 and 2	Topical therapy is not effective. Systemic acyclovir or valacyclovir
Shingles or disseminated herpes zoster	Varicella zoster virus	Systemic acyclovir or valacyclovir. Choose the oral or IV route according to severity

Abbreviations: CA-MRSA, community-acquired MRSA; MSSA, methicillin-susceptible *Staphylococcus aureus*; MRSA, methicillin-resistant *Staphylococcus aureus*; TMP/SMX, trimethoprim/ sulfamethoxazole.

Laboratory tests

- Gram stain and wound cultures are not useful in patients with cellulitis. If abscesses, ulcers, or open wounds are present, wound cultures are relevant for bacterial identification and treatment selection.
- Blood cultures are relevant to confirm diagnosis when cellulitis with systemic compromise is suspected. Complete blood count (CBC) and differential and C-reactive protein may be useful to assess systemic compromise and to follow treatment response.

Management for Patients with Years of Life Expectancy

- Antibiotics should be selected according to suspected microorganisms, clinical judgment, and laboratory tests. Antimicrobial therapy should be chosen according to the site and extent of infection, bacterial susceptibility, available administration routes, renal and hepatic function, drug interactions, and costs (Table 36.2).
- General management including IV fluids and hospital/ICU admission should be considered according to the severity of the disease. Manage pain with acetaminophen, nonsteroidal antiinflammatory drugs (NSAIDs), or opioids as appropriate.
- Wound care is not necessary for the management of cellulitis or erysipelas, unless ulcers, abscesses, or open wounds are present. Surgical debridement for necrotizing fasciitis, diabetic foot, and deep pressure ulcers should be promptly performed when required.
- Identification of skin breakdowns, such as interdigital mycosis, dry skin, pressure ulcers, subcutaneous or intravenous devices, or tumor-related skin erosions, should be actively sought to identify risk factors for repeated skin

Table 36.2 First Line Antibiotics and Dosing for Cellulitis and Erysipelas

Infection	Antibiotic	Route	Dosing*
Cellulitis and erysipelas	Penicillin G	IV	1–2 million IU q6h
	Cefazolin	IV	1 g q8h
	Vancomycin	IV	15 mg/kg q12h (if allergic to ONC or cefazolin)
	Cefadroxil	PO	500 mg–1 g q12h
	Doxycylin	PO	100 mg BID
	TMP-SMX	PO	1 double strength tablet q8–12 h
	Dicloxacillin	PO	500 mg QID
	Clindamycin	PO	300 mg TID

*The usual treatment duration is 7–14 days. Consider switching from IV to PO when the patient is afebrile. Consider starting treatment through the PO route if there is no systemic compromise and in the outpatient setting.

infections and for prevention. Prevention with daily skin care, including moisturizing and hydration, nutritional support, and mobility, is important in all patients.

Relevance to the Cancer Palliative Care Setting

- Cancer patients may be at higher risk of cellulitis due to disruption of the skin as a result of wounds, inflammation, use of subcutaneous or intravenous devices, lymphedema, and systemic abnormalities such as neutropenia or cachexia.
- Consider a wide differential diagnosis as both the underlying disease and cancer treatments may have skin manifestations that can mimic skin infections (e.g., Sweet syndrome, radiation dermatitis, or epidermal growth factor receptor inhibitor-induced folliculitis).
- Cancer patients undergoing systemic chemotherapy who develop skin infections may be at higher risk of complications due to neutropenia. Consider widening the antimicrobial therapy spectrum according to specific risk factors.
- Patients with advanced cancer may be at higher risk of pressure ulcers due to impaired mobility and cachexia. Active prevention is essential.

Management for Patients with Months of Life Expectancy

- Management is similar to patients with years of life expectancy. Treatment with antibiotics is generally indicated based on guidelines and adapted according to clinical judgment. Surgical procedures may be considered assessing individual surgical risk, possible benefits, and patient prognosis.

Management for Patients with Weeks/Days of Life Expectancy

- There are no available evidence-based guidelines on the use of antibiotics in palliative care patients.
- Local lesions should be managed as usual. The interventions are usually simple and nonexpensive and can easily provide patients with symptom relief.
- Patient prognosis, patient's symptoms, wishes and values, and feasibility of IV antibiotic therapy should be considered when managing patients with severe skin infections at home. In a small study of home care patients with infections, 41% of those who had skin or subcutaneous infections had reduction of fever and/or amelioration of symptoms within 3 days of antibiotic use.
- Surgical management should not be considered in patients with a short-term prognosis. Wound care and systemic analgesia should always be implemented if needed.

- Patients at the end of life may have their oral route impaired. These patients can use the subcutaneous route for antibiotic administration and hydration. With the subcutaneous route, it is important to frequently assess for skin infection or irritation close to the needle injection site.
- Consider local or systemic antibiotic use (e.g., metronidazole) for infected malodorous wounds.

Recommended Reading

1. Berger TG. *Dermatologic Disorders in Current Medical Diagnosis and Treatment (51st ed.)*. McGraw-Hill, New York, 2012.

2. Kofteridis DP, Valachis A, Koutsounaki E, Maraki S. Skin and soft tissue infections in patients with solid tumours. *Scient World J* 2012;2012:804518.

3. Gilbert DN. *The Sanford Guide to Antimicrobial Therapy*. Antimicrobial Therapy, Incorporated, Sperryville, VA, 2013.

4. Mandell GL, Bennett JE, Dolin R. *Mandell, Douglas, and Bennett's Principles and Practice of Infectious Diseases*. Churchill Livingstone/Elsevier, St. Louis, MO, 2010

5. Nakagawa S, Toya Y, Okamoto Y, et al. Can anti-infective drugs improve the infection-related symptoms of patients with cancer during the terminal stages of their lives? *J Palliative Med* 2010;13(5):535–540.

6. Reinbolt RE, Shenk AM, White PH, Navari RM. Symptomatic treatment of infections in patients with advanced cancer receiving hospice care. *J Pain Symptom Manage* 2005;30(2):175–182.

Chapter 37

Herpes Infections

Linh Nguyen

Common Viral Infections

- Herpes simplex virus type 1 and 2 (HSV-1 and HSV-2)
- Varicella zoster virus (VZV)—Primary (chicken pox), reactivation (herpes zoster or shingles), disseminated
- Cytomegalovirus (CMV)
- Human herpes virus 6 (HHV-6)
- Epstein–Barr virus (EBV)

Symptoms and Signs

- HSV—Cold sores (oral pain, dysphagia, dyspepsia; on examination yellowish lesions are easily removed from mucosa, vesicles on lips, or "cold sores"); esophagitis (retrosternal pain); chronic localized ulcers on the nose, lips, or eyelids; localized lesions on genitals and perianal areas; may disseminate widely.
- VZV—Chicken pox (pediatric patients, generalized vesicular rash and fever, starts on the face/scalp spreading to the trunk/extremities, new lesions and older crusted lesions); herpes zoster (pain, unilateral vesicular rash in dermatomal distribution, postherpetic neuralgia with zoster-associated pain >1 month).
- CMV—Pneumonia and gastroenteritis are most common; other infections include esophagitis, myocarditis, hepatitis, encephalitis, and retinitis.
- HHV-6—Fever, rash, pneumonitis, hepatitis, myelosuppression, and neurologic dysfunction mainly in transplant patients. Common in pediatric patients.
- EBV—Mononucleosis-like syndrome (fever, sore throat, lymphadenopathy) and posttransplant lymphoproliferative disorders; dissemination can occur from localized nodular lesions.

Investigations

- HSV—Mainly a clinical diagnosis and should be differentiated from aphthous ulcers. Herpetic vesicles precede ulcers, are located on hard gingiva or hard palate, and appear as crops of lesions. Direct fluorescent antibody, viral culture, polymerase chain reaction (PCR), evidence of viropathic changes on biopsy, and exfoliative cytology can be used to confirm the diagnosis. Anti-HSV IgG antibody testing should be performed in patients with acute leukemias on induction chemotherapy or allogeneic hematopoietic stem cell transplantation recipients because seropositive individuals should receive acyclovir prophylaxis to prevent reactivation. Type-specific anti-HSV IgG serology testing is not necessary.

- VZV—Laboratory confirmation is not required; direct fluorescent antibody, viral culture, PCR, or evidence of viropathic changes on biopsy. Vesicles on nasal tip or side indicate nasociliary branch involvement and an ophthalmology referral is recommended to exclude orbital involvement.
- CMV—Early detection is critical to management. CMV pp65 antigenemia assay of infected white blood cells (WBC) or serum real-time polymerase chain reaction should be considered.
- HHV-6—Routine testing is not recommended.
- EBV—Clinical diagnosis (triad of fever, pharyngitis, and lymphadenopathy for 1 to 4 weeks), moderately elevated WBC count, increased total number of lymphocytes, >10% atypical lymphocytes, and positive "monospot" test.

Relevance to the Cancer Palliative Care Setting

- Herpes infection may contribute to symptom burden and can cause significant pain, dysphagia, and dyspepsia. Secondary infection with bacteria and fungi may occur. Zoster may contribute to morbidity if postherpetic neuralgia occurs. Widespread dissemination to the lungs, liver, and central nervous system (CNS) is potentially life threatening.
- CMV, HHV-6, and EBV are important pathogens in stem cell transplant patients.

Management for Patients with Years of Life Expectancy

- HSV—Oral infections should be treated with acyclovir orally or intravenously; maintain hydration and monitor renal function. Treat concurrent infections and maintain oral hygiene. Chlorhexidine (0.2% twice daily rinsing) may be beneficial in HSV-1 infections. When extraoral lesions become secondarily infected, topical antibiotics are indicated. In patients with radiotherapy-induced or chemotherapy-induced stomatitis who are seropositive and myelosuppressed, topical and systemic acyclovir is effective. Seropositive patients receiving selected chemotherapy or undergoing stem cell transplantation patients should receive prophylaxis with acyclovir. Acyclovir, famciclovir, and valacyclovir are effective for disseminated infections (Table 37.1).
- VZV—Oral famciclovir and valacyclovir are more effective than acyclovir in cancer patients. VZV treatment shortens viral shedding, accelerates

Table 37.1 Typical Medications and Doses for Viral Infections

Class	Common Medications and Doses
Anti-herpes simplex virus (HSV)	Acyclovir 5 mg/kg/dose IV every 8 h for 7 days (up to 14 days also reported)
Mucocutaneous	Acyclovir 400 mg PO 5 times daily for 7 days (unlabeled use)
Orolabial	Acyclovir topical: ½-inch ribbon of ointment for a 4-inch square surface area every 3 h (6 times/day) for 7 days
	Acyclovir 200–400 mg PO 5 times daily for 5 days for episodic/recurrent treatment
	Acyclovir 200 mg PO 5 times daily or 400 mg 3 times daily for 7–10 days for initial treatment has been recommended by some clinicians
	Acyclovir topical: apply 5 times/day for 4 days
Anti-varicella zoster virus (VZV) (shingles)	Famciclovir 500 mg PO every 8 h for 7 days
	Valacyclovir 1 g PO 3 times daily for 7 days

healing of lesions, and reduces the frequency of visceral disease. Severe infections (meningoencephalitis, pneumonitis) require IV acyclovir. Administer varicella-zoster immune globulin for postexposure prophylaxis in high-risk patients, which can also ameliorate established infection.

- CMV—Ganciclovir is the usual therapy. Monitor for neutropenia, which is the dose-limiting toxicity.
- HHV-6—Ganciclovir and foscarnet inhibit *in vitro* viral replication. Clinical experience is minimal.
- EBV—Reduce immunosuppressive therapy if possible. Rituximab is recommended for posttransplant lymphoproliferative disorders.

Management for Patients with Months of Life Expectancy

- Herpes management is similar to patients with years of life expectancy.
- For patients with advanced cancer and HSV infections the oral and topical routes (5% acyclovir) are better palliative options, especially if the patient is able to swallow.

Management for Patients with Weeks/Days of Life Expectancy

- At the end of life, patients may not be able to swallow. Therefore the topical route is preferred.

Recommended Reading

1. De Conno F, Martini C, Sbanotto A, et al. *Oxford Textbook of Palliative Medicine (4th ed.).* Oxford University Press, Oxford, England, 2010: 996–1014.

2. Rolston KVI, Bodey GF. Infections in patients with cancer. In Kufe DW, Frei E, Holland JF, et al. (eds.). *Holland-Frei Cancer Medicine* (8th ed.). People's Medical Publishing House-USA, Shelton, CT, 2010: 1921–1940.

3. Eguia JM. Infectious disease. In Le T, Chin-Hong P, Baudendistel TE, Rubinson L (eds.). *First Aid for the Internal Medicine Boards*. McGraw-Hill, New York, 2006: 395–400.

4. Centers for Disease Control and Prevention. Infectious Disease Society of America., American Society of Blood and Marrow Transplantation: Guidelines for preventing opportunistic infections among hematopoietic stem cell transplant recipients. *MMWR Recommend Rep* 2000;49 (RR-10):1–125, CE1-7.

Chapter 38

Fungal Infections

Linh Nguyen

Common Organisms

- *Candida*
- *Aspergillus*
- *Cryptococcus*

Symptoms and Signs

- *Candida*
  - Intertrigo ("diaper rash")—Pruritic vesiculopustules rupture to form macerated or fissured beefy-red areas at skin folds; satellite lesions may be present.
  - Oral thrush—Oral pain, burning sensation of tongue or mucosa, white-yellowish plaques, easily wiped off, leaving a bleeding painful surface.
  - Candidal esophagitis—Dysphagia, odynophagia, retrosternal chest pain.
  - Candidemia and disseminated candidiasis—No characteristic symptoms/signs; may have an acute onset of tachycardia, tachypnea, hypotension, and fever unresponsive to antibiotics. Ocular infection (with eye pain, blurred vision, scotomata, or loss of visual acuity), osteomyelitis, arthritis, or endocarditis may occur. Erythematous macronodular skin lesions sometimes associated with myositis may be seen.
  - Hepatosplenic candidiasis—Fever and abdominal pain emerge as neutropenia resolves following bone marrow transplantation.
- *Aspergillus*—Fever; lung infection (pneumonia, hemorrhage, infarction, abscesses, bronchitis); sinoorbital infection (retroorbital pain, headache, circumorbital erythema, nasal obstruction, necrotic encrustation of the nasal septum, palate, external nares); may invade the brain or destruct paranasal/facial structures and eyes; may disseminate widely to other organs resulting in abscess, thrombosis, and/or infarction; central nervous system (CNS) involvement (lethargy, focal neurologic signs); skin lesions; stomatitis.
- *Cryptococcus*—Meningoencephalitis (headache, vertigo, nausea, vomiting; signs of fever, meningitis, stupor, increased intracranial pressure, focal neurologic defects); atypical pneumonia.

Investigations

- *Candida*
  - Oral thrush—Clinical diagnosis by appearance or scraping with KOH (potassium hydroxide) preparation or Gram stain
  - Candidal esophagitis—Endoscopic appearance of white patches or biopsy showing mucosal invasion. May have a cobblestone or moth-eaten appearance of the esophageal mucosa on a barium-swallow study
  - Candidemia and disseminated candidiasis—Cultures of blood, body fluids, or aspirates
  - Hepatosplenic candidiasis—Ultrasound or computed tomography (CT) imaging showing abscesses
- *Aspergillus*
  - High-resolution CT scanning of the lungs for patients with normal chest radiographs, CT scan of sinuses, nasal cultures, pathologic examination, and culture from biopsy in sinoorbital infections. Galactomannan assay and polymerase chain reaction (PCR) are promising.
- *Cryptococcus*—CT or magnetic resonance imaging (MRI), lumbar puncture, fungal culture

Relevance to the Cancer Palliative Care Setting

- Cancer patients are at risk of fungal infections secondary to chemotherapy, steroids, surgical procedures, and instrumentation. Patients with acute leukemia and hematopoietic stem cell transplant recipients are at particularly high risk of developing invasive fungal infections and often need antifungal prophylaxis (e.g., fluconazole, itraconazole, posaconazole).
- Patients with advanced cancer often receive repeated courses of antifungal medications for recurrent fungal infections. Therefore, azole resistance may emerge.
- Fungal infections may contribute to symptom burden and can cause significant pain, dysphagia, and anorexia.
- Fungal infections may complicate radiotherapy-induced and chemotherapy-induced stomatitis.
- Opioids (methadone and fentanyl) and antifungals drug–drug interactions should be considered. Azole antifungals can increase methadone levels and cause toxicity.

Management for Patients with Years of Life Expectancy (see Table 38.1)

- *Candida*
  - Intertrigo—Topical antifungals (nystatin, clotrimazole, miconazole creams)
  - Oral thrush—Nystatin suspension swish and swallow is the classic treatment but is not always effective. An alternative is ice lollies made of

Table 38.1 Typical Medications and Doses for Fungal Infections

Class	Common Medications and Doses
Intertrigo	Nystatin topical: apply 2–3 times/day to affected areas; very moist topical lesions are best treated with powder
Oropharyngeal/ thrush	Clotrimazole topical: apply to affected area twice daily (morning and evening) for 7 consecutive days Fluconazole 200 mg PO/IV on day 1; maintenance dose 100 mg IV daily for ≥ 2 weeks (manufacturer's recommendation) Fluconazole 100–200 mg PO/IV daily for 7–14 days for uncomplicated, moderate-to-severe disease; chronic therapy of 100 mg IV 3 times weekly is recommended in immunocompromised patients with a history of oropharyngeal candidiasis (alternative dosing) Itraconazole 100–200 mg PO once daily for a minimum of 3 weeks; continue dosing for 2 weeks after resolution of symptoms Nystatin suspension (swish and swallow) 400,000–600,000 units 4 times/day; swish in the mouth and retain for as long as possible (several minutes) before swallowing Clotrimazole lozenge: 10 mg troche dissolved slowly 5 times/day for 14 consecutive days
Candidal esophagitis	Fluconazole 200 mg PO/IV on day 1, then maintenance dose of 100–400 mg daily for 21 days and for at least 2 weeks following the resolution of symptoms (manufacturer's recommendation) Fluconazole 200–400 mg PO/IV daily for 12–21 days; suppressive therapy of 100–200 mg 3 times weekly may be used for recurrent infections (alternative dosing)

nystatin diluted with water. A combination with chlorhexidine reduces nystatin activity. Other topicals that include clotrimazole and miconazole lozenges may be considered. In severe cases, both topical and systemic therapy such as fluconazole and itraconazole can be used together.

- Esophagitis and other deep or disseminated infections—Fluconazole is generally effective for esophagitis. Other options include amphotericin, voriconazole, and caspofungin.
- *Candida* colonization in the sputum and urine should be treated in patients with surgery or abnormalities of the genitourinary (GU) tract, neutropenia, or diabetes mellitus due to the risk of serious *Candida* infection.
- *Aspergillus*—Voriconazole is the agent of choice. Surgical resection of a residual cavity should be considered due to reactivation; patients with residual lesions and neutropenia should be treated with antifungals.
- *Cryptococcus*—Amphotericin B + 5-fluorocytosine for 2 weeks followed by fluconazole for at least 10 weeks.

Management for Patients with Months of Life Expectancy

- Management is similar to patients with years of life expectancy.

Management for Patients with Weeks/Days of Life Expectancy

- At the end of life, patients may not be able to swallow.
- Lozenges, ice lollies, IV routes, and once daily medications should be considered for patients with oral thrush who can benefit from treatment.
- Prophylactic antifungals may be of limited benefit in this setting although no studies have been conducted in this population.

Recommended Reading

1. Rolston KVI, Bodey GF. Infections in patients with cancer. In Kufe DW, Frei E, Holland JF, et al. (eds.). *Holland-Frei Cancer Medicine* (8th ed.). People's Medical Publishing House-USA, Shelton, CT, 2010: 1921–1940.

2. Eguia JM. Infectious disease. In Le T, Chin-Hong P, Baudendistel TE, Rubinson L (eds.). *First Aid for the Internal Medicine Boards.* McGraw-Hill, New York, 2006: 395–400.

3. De Conno F, Martini C, Sbanotto A, et al. *Oxford Textbook of Palliative Medicine (4th ed.).* Oxford University Press, Oxford, England, 2010: 996–1014.

Section VIII

Endocrine

Chapter 39

Diabetes

Kunal C. Kadakia and Rony Dev

Classification

- Diabetes mellitus Type I (DMI)—approximately 10% of cases
  - Also referred to as juvenile or insulin-dependent diabetes mellitus
  - Diagnosed in childhood or early adulthood
  - Due to immunologic destruction of pancreatic β cells → eventually to the complete absence of insulin secretion
- Diabetes mellitus Type II (DMII)—approximately 90% of cases
  - Also referred to as adult-onset or non-insulin-dependent diabetes mellitus.
  - DMII often becomes insulin dependent due to β-cell exhaustion in the setting of chronic insulin resistance after approximately 7–10 years.
  - It is diagnosed in adults and is associated with obesity.
  - It is related to reduced sensitivity to insulin at peripheral insulin receptors → increased endogenous insulin secretion and subsequent insulin requirement.
- Secondary hyperglycemia
  - Cancer—Multifactorial; secondary to insulin resistance, aberrant counterregulatory hormone production (i.e., growth hormone), poor skeletal muscle glucose utilization, and increased hepatic glucose production
  - Medications—Glucocorticoids (most often with previously undiagnosed DM), thiazide diuretics, amphetamines (i.e., methylphenidate), excess thyroid supplementation, phenytoin
  - Systemic Inflammation—Infection/sepsis, trauma, pancreatitis, postsurgical
  - Pancreatic insufficiency—Pancreatitis, hemochromatosis, cystic fibrosis, postresection

Symptoms and Signs

- Hyperglycemic—Osmotic diuresis (present when plasma glucose is >180–200 mg/dL, the renal glucose threshold) can cause dehydration, polyuria, and polydipsia. It is associated with weight loss, poor wound healing, and recurrent infections. Diabetic ketoacidosis (DKA) and hyperglycemic hyperosmolar state (HHS) can also occur (see Table 39.1). Signs of volume depletion include decreased skin turgor, xerostomia, hypotension, somnolence, and delirium.
- Hypoglycemic (secondary to diabetic medications)—Symptoms include tremors, anxiety, lethargy, palpitations, seizures, and coma. Signs include diaphoresis, tachycardia, somnolence, and delirium.

Table 39.1 Clinical Characteristics of Hyperglycemic Hyperosmolar State and Diabetic Ketoacidosis

	Hyperosmolar Nonketotic Syndrome (HONK)	Diabetic Ketoacidosis (DKA)
Patient characteristics	Due to severe dehydration secondary to osmotic diuresis. Most often in older patients with DMII. Follows acute stressors (i.e., infection) and develops subacutely (days to weeks).	Due to lack of insulin. Almost always in DMI following acute stressor (i.e., infection, glucocorticoids, ischemia, failure to take insulin) and develops acutely (hours to days).
Clinical manifestations	Polyuria, polydipsia, weight loss, delirium, coma, seizures	Polyuria, polydipsia, nausea/vomiting, abdominal pain, ileus, delirium, Kussmaul's respirations (deep breaths with odor of acetone)
Laboratory findings	Serum glucose >600 mg/dL, serum osmolality (>320 mOsm/L), ↑ BUN and Cr, usually no ketoacidosis	Serum glucose 200–600 mg/dL, ↑ urine/plasma ketones, acidosis, ↑ anion gap
Treatment*	Aggressive hydration (average fluid loss of 8–10 L) followed by insulin (0.05–0.1 U/kg/h followed by SQ insulin)	Insulin (0.1 U/kg/h continuous until anion gap normalizes, followed by SQ insulin), aggressive hydration, electrolyte repletion

* Consult endocrinology expert if needed.
Abbreviations: Cr, creatinine; DMI, diabetes mellitus Type I; DMII, diabetes mellitus Type II; BUN, blood urea nitrogen.

Investigations

- Diagnosis of diabetes—Fasting glucose >126 mg/dL on two occasions, random glucose >200 mg/dL with hyperglycemic symptoms, $Hb_{A1c} \geq 6.5$, or administration of a 75 g oral glucose tolerance test with 2-hour value >200 mg/dL on two occasions.
- Target fasting glucose is based on goals of care (up to 180–220 mg/dL). No consensus agreement exists.
- Glucose monitoring should be tailored to the specific palliative care population (see below).

Relevance to the Cancer Palliative Care Setting

- Diabetes is common in cancer patients.
- Symptomatic hypoglycemia can occur due to complications of cancer including erratic oral intake, anorexia/cachexia, and renal/liver insufficiency.
- Therapy with glucocorticoids can lead to symptomatic hyperglycemia.
- Hyperglycemia may increase the risk of infections and impair wound healing in cancer patients. Both hypoglycemia and hyperglycemia may contribute to delirium.

Management for Patients with Years of Life Expectancy

- Knowledge of the pharmacopeia related to diabetes care in the palliative care patient can reduce the incidence of symptomatic hypoglycemia (see Table 39.2).
- General—Begin discussions regarding reducing the need for intense glycemic control. Educate regarding signs of hypoglycemia, though hypoglycemic unawareness is common in older patients with comorbidities.

Table 39.2 Common Diabetic Medications

Medication Class	Examples	General Comments	Dose Adjustments
Insulin Rapid-acting Intermediate Long-acting	Lispro, aspart NPH Glargine, detemir	Simplest regimen should be used. Usually requires combination of long-acting basal insulin as well as rapid-acting mealtime coverage. If erratic oral intake, can give a rapid-acting dose immediately after meal.	Decreased metabolism of insulin with renal/liver insufficiency. Dose must be reduced. Adjust dose based on oral intake.
Biguanides	Metformin	Low risk of hypoglycemia. GI distress common. Can be anorexigenic.	Discontinue in renal/liver insufficiency due to rare but serious lactic acidosis.
Sulfonylureas	Glyburide, glipizide, glimepiride	All are long-acting with active metabolites except glipizide, which has less risk of prolonged hypoglycemia.	Discontinue in renal/liver insufficiency. Adjust dose based on oral intake.
Thiazolidinediones	Pioglitazone, rosiglitazone	Low risk of hypoglycemia. Leads to fluid retention and edema.	Discontinue in liver insufficiency. Avoid in heart disease as it can cause heart failure.
Meglitinides	Repaglinide, nateflinide	Due to rapid onset and preprandial dosing can be used for postprandial hyperglycemia if oral intake is erratic.	Discontinue in renal/liver insufficiency. Adjust dose based on oral intake.
α-Glucosidase inhibitors	Acarbose	Gastrointestinal distress is common (bloating). Low risk for hypoglycemia as dosed prandial.	Discontinue if there is no oral intake.
Dipeptidyl peptidase-4 (DPP-IV) inhibitor	Saxagliptin, sitagliptin	Nausea is common. Can cause acute pancreatitis.	Adjust dose in renal insufficiency. Discontinue if nausea is present.
Glucagon-like receptor-1 (GLP-1) agonists	Pramlintide, exenatide	Nausea and weight loss are common. Can cause acute pancreatitis.	Discontinue in renal insufficiency or if nausea/anorexia is present.

- Type I diabetes—Patients require both long or intermediate acting insulin such as glargine for basal insulin needs and preprandial rapid-acting insulin for mealtime coverage. If oral intake is reduced or erratic, can give rapid-acting insulin dose immediately after meal if the patient eats or omit the dose if the patient does not eat. Continue checking fasting glucose as often as necessary to maintain euglycemia.

- Type II diabetes—Patients often continue with previous oral hypoglycemic or insulin regimen. If nausea, anorexia, or erratic oral intake occurs, reduce or discontinue oral hypoglycemic (see Table 39.2). Reduce or discontinue glucose monitoring unless symptoms suggest poor glycemic control.

Management for Patients with Months of Life Expectancy

- Management is similar to patients with years of life expectancy. Adjust insulin doses based on renal/liver insufficiency.

- Type I diabetes—Maintain both long-acting basal insulin and preprandial rapid-acting insulin for mealtime coverage (see above). Due to weight loss or poor oral intake, patients will require an insulin dose less than earlier in the course of illness. The goal for glycemic control should be less stringent. Continue glucose checks as previously if physically able with an aim to focus on avoidance of symptomatic hypoglycemia or hyperglycemia.

- Type II diabetes—Advise patients to reduce or stop oral hypoglycemic and insulin regimen (specifically, insulin and sulfonylureas due to high incidence of hypoglycemia). Advise pleasure-based diet. Decrease or stop glucose monitoring unless symptoms of hypoglycemia or hyperglycemia occur.

Management for Patients with Weeks/Days of Life Expectancy

- For symptomatic hypoglycemia—Give 3–5 tablets of dextrose if oral intake is possible. If only PEG access, can use 150 mL of nondiet cola. If there is no enteral access, give 1 mg glucagon intramuscularly (can be ineffective in liver disease). If there is IV access, can give 75 mL of 20% glucose over 10 minutes.

- Weeks of life expectancy—For type II diabetes, stop all oral hypoglycemics and decrease the insulin dose. In type I diabetes, decrease the insulin dose and consider switching to an intermediate-acting (NPH) or rapid-acting regimen and adjust the insulin dose based on renal/liver insufficiency. Continue to educate patients and families regarding the reduced need for glycemic control and monitor for symptoms of hypoglycemia.

- At the end of life, avoid glucose checks if possible. Abandoning glucose monitoring completely could lead to patient and family distress. As such, discussions should focus on the importance of minimizing harm and maintaining comfort rather than "futility."

Recommended Reading

1. Angelo M, Ruchalski C, Sproge BJ. An approach to diabetes mellitus in hospice and palliative medicine. *J Palliat Med* 2011;14(1):83–87.

2. Budge P. Management of diabetes in patients at the end of life. *Nurs Stand* 2010;25(6):42–46.

3. King EJ, Haboubi H, Evans D, Baker I, Bain SC, Stephens JW. The management of diabetes in terminal illness related to cancer. *QJM* 2012;100(1):3–9.

Chapter 40

Hyperthyroidism

Kunal C. Kadakia and Rony Dev

Classification

- Primary hyperthyroidism
  - Graves' Disease (diffuse toxic goiter)—Most common type; ≈90%.
    - Autoimmune disorder caused by abnormal IgG antibody binding to thyroid-stimulating hormone (TSH) receptors.
    - Most commonly affects women 20–50 years of age.
  - Toxic multinodular goiter and toxic thyroid adenoma—Unknown etiologies, related to activating mutations in TSH receptor genes. Presence of both normal and abnormal autonomously functioning thyroid tissue is pathognomonic. It is more common in older adults.
- Subacute thyroiditis
  - Granulomatous thyroiditis—Also known as de Quervain's thyroiditis or classic painful thyroiditis. It is generally secondary to viral illness such as mumps and coxsackievirus.
  - Silent thyroiditis—Painless thyroiditis. An autoimmune condition with antithyroid antibodies (lower titers than in Hashimoto's thyroiditis).
  - Postpartum thyroiditis—Occurs after 5–10% of pregnancies.
- Nonthyroidal disease
  - Exogenous thyrotoxicosis—Iatrogenic or factitious
  - Pharmacologic—Excessive iodine ingestion (Jod–Basedow effect), amiodarone, interferon
  - Malignancy (rare)—TSH production by pituitary tumors, autonomous thyroid hormone production by teratomas of the ovary (struma ovarii), metastatic thyroid cancer

Symptoms and Signs

- Symptoms—Palpitations, fine tremor, restlessness, fatigue, nervousness, heat intolerance, weakness, diarrhea, insomnia, and amenorrhea/oligomenorrhea. In addition, weight loss and depression can be seen in elderly patients ("apathetic thyrotoxicosis").
- Signs—Tachycardia, hypertension, arrhythmia (atrial fibrillation or premature ventricular contractions), wide pulse pressure, lid lag and exophthalmos (only in Graves' disease), thyroid bruit, proximal muscle weakness, and brisk deep tendon reflexes.

- Thyroid storm can be present with exaggerated symptoms and signs as described above with psychosis, agitation, volume overload, delirium, fever, stupor, or coma.

Investigations

- Thyroid function tests—TSH, free T_4, and free T_3 are all useful for diagnosis. In nearly all cases, TSH is low and free T_3 and T_4 are elevated (i.e., Graves' disease). Low TSH with normal free T_3 and T_4 suggests subclinical hyperthyroidism, generally asymptomatic. Low TSH with low free T_4 and sometimes low free T_4 suggests sick euthyroid syndrome.
- 24-hour radioactive iodine uptake (RAIU) and scan—Can help distinguish between increased release of preformed thyroid hormone (decreased uptake, such as in thyroiditis) from excessive endogenous production of thyroid hormone (high uptake, such as in Graves' disease).
- Other tests—Thyroid-stimulating antibodies and antithyroid antibodies can be positive in Graves' disease. Glucose intolerance and hyperlipidemia can be observed.

Relevance to the Cancer Palliative Care Setting

- Hyperthyroidism may occur as a result of cancer treatments such as radiation leading to radiation thyroiditis or drug-induced thyroiditis from sunitinib or interferon-α (rare).
- Rarely, metastatic follicular carcinoma with bone metastases can be associated with symptoms of hyperthyroidism.

Management for Patients with Years of Life Expectancy (see Table 40.1)

- Medical Management—Medical therapy consists of alleviating the adrenergic manifestations of thyrotoxicosis with β-blockers and reducing the synthesis of thyroid hormones with thionamides.
  - Any β-blocker can be used and titrated to symptomatic relief; consider atenolol 25–50 mg/daily (up to 200 mg/daily) given the advantage of β_1 selectivity and once daily dosing.
  - Thionamides include propylthiouracil (PTU) and methimazole. Methimazole is most often used (initial dose of 30–40 mg/daily) given its advantage over PTU due to once daily dosing, more rapid induction of a euthyroid state, less effect on success of subsequent radioactive iodine, and less hepatotoxicity. PTU is used during the first trimester of pregnancy due to the teratogenicity of methimazole. Skin toxicity is common (~10–15%); monitor for hepatotoxicity and agranulocytosis (rare). Treatment is tapered to the lowest dose to maintain euthyroidism and after 1–2 years can be discontinued as permanent remission is possible.

Table 40.1 Hyperthyroidism and Associated Diagnostic Testing					
	TSH	**fT4**	**fT3**	**RAIU**	**Exam**
Graves' Disease	↓	↑	↑	↑ (Diffuse)	Diffuse Goiter
Thyroiditis	↓	N/↑	N/↑	↓ (Diffuse)	Tender in subacute; nontender in silent
Toxic multinodular goiter/adenoma	↓	N/↑	N/↑	↑ (Nodular)	Nodule(s)
Exogenous thyrotoxicosis	↓	↑	↑	↓	Normal
Pituitary Adenoma	N/↑	↑	↑	↑	Minimal Goiter
Subclinical Hyperthyroidism	↓	N	N	↑/↓	Variable

- Radioactive iodine (RAI)—Most often used in Graves' disease; can be used in toxic nodular goiter and toxic adenoma.
  - One dose of iodine-131 can lead to a euthyroid state in 75% of patients with Graves' disease. It is more common now to target for posttreatment hypothyroidism to reduce treatment failure rates.
  - Major advantages include the avoidance of surgery and need for thionamides.
  - Disadvantages include worsening of Graves' eyes disease and the development of permanent hypothyroidism requiring replacement therapy.
- Subtotal or total thyroidectomy—Leads to rapid cure of hyperthyroidism (after antithyroid drugs have induced a euthyroid state).
  - Disadvantages include the development of permanent hypothyroidism (even with subtotal resection), recurrent laryngeal nerve injury, hypoparathyroidism, and the need for anesthesia and hospitalization.
- Thyroiditis—Subacute thyroiditis is self-limited and treatment is symptomatic with β-blockers and nonsteroidal drugs. Silent thyroiditis is also self-limited and treatment is symptomatic with β-blockers if needed.
  - Toxic nodular goiter and toxic adenoma—RAI is commonly used as it often ablates toxic nodule and renders the patient euthyroid afterward. It can also be treated with thyroidectomy or removal of toxic adenoma.
  - Thyroid storm—Consult an endocrinology expert emergently. A combination of β-blockers, corticosteroids, and thioamides is most often used. β-Blockers are used with caution in the setting of congestive heart failure.

Management for Patients with Months of Life Expectancy

- Management is similar to patients with years of life expectancy.

Management for Patients with Weeks/Days of Life Expectancy

- No data exist on the prevalence of symptomatic hyperthyroidism in patients receiving palliative care.

- At the end of life, patients may not be able to swallow. Intravenous β-blockers can be used to alleviate adverse symptoms of thyrotoxicosis. Avoid frequent blood work if possible.

Recommended Reading

1. Grossmann M, Premaratne E, Desai J, Davis ID. Thyrotoxicosis during sunitinib treatment for renal cell carcinoma. *Clin Endocrinol* 2008;69(4):669–672.

2. Klein I, Becker DV, Levey GS. Treatment of hyperthyroid disease. *Ann Intern Med* 1994;121(4):281–288.

Chapter 41

Hypothyroidism

David Hui

Classification

- Primary hypothyroidism
  - Thyroiditis—Hashimoto's, subacute, irradiation, postpartum
  - Iatrogenic—Thyroidectomy, radioactive ^{131}I
  - Medications—Methimazole, propylthiouracil, iodide, lithium, amiodarone
  - Others—Iodine deficiency, thyroid agenesis, thyroid dysgenesis, idiopathic
- Secondary hypothyroidism (central causes)—Tumor, infiltration, infarction, infection, surgery, and/or irradiation of the pituitary/hypothalamus

Symptoms and Signs

- Symptoms—Fatigue, dry skin, cold intolerance, goiter, depression, confusion, decreased memory, constipation, weakness, carpel tunnel syndrome, menorrhagia, amenorrhea, and weight gain
- Signs—Bradycardia, bradypnea, diastolic hypertension, hypothermia, cool and dry skin, vitiligo, orange skin (from carotonemia), carpel tunnel syndrome, hair thinning, periorbital edema, anemia, goiter, pleural effusion, pericardial effusion, nonpitting edema, proximal myopathy, pseudomyotonia, and hyporeflexia

Investigations

- Thyroid-stimulating hormone (TSH) is usually the only test required to make a diagnosis of hypothyroidism. Free T_4 and free T_3 are not generally needed unless secondary hypothyroidism is suspected (Table 41.1).
- Anti-thyroid peroxidase (TPO) antibodies and anti-thyroglobulin antibodies may be useful if Hashimoto's thyroiditis is suspected.

Relevance to the Cancer Palliative Care Setting

- Hypothyroidism may occur as a result of cancer treatments such as thyroidectomy, previous head and neck radiation, and various targeted agents such as sorafenib and sunitinib.
- Hypothyroidism may contribute to symptom burden and can cause significant fatigue, drowsiness, constipation, and/or depressed mood. In patients

Table 41.1 Hypothyroidism and Laboratory Findings

	Thyroid-Stimulating Hormone (TSH)	Free T₃	Free T₄
Primary hypothyroidism	↑	↓	↓
Secondary hypothyroidism	↓	↓	↓
Sick euthyroid syndrome	Normal/↑/↓	↓	Normal/↓
Subclinical hypothyroidism	↑	Normal	Normal

with these symptoms and a reasonable life expectancy, screening for hypothyroidism may be warranted. Hypothyroidism may also be associated with delirium and, in severe cases, with myxedema coma.

Management for Patients with Years of Life Expectancy

- Thyroid replacement therapy—Levothyroxine (T₄) 75–100 µg PO daily (1.6 µg/kg/day). Initiate treatment at a lower dose (25–50 µg daily and titrate up by 25 µg per month) in the elderly or those with risk factors for heart disease. It takes approximately 6–8 weeks for TSH to equilibrate after each thyroid medication adjustment.
- Subclinical hypothyroidism—Consider initiating treatment if the patient is symptomatic or has a positive antithyroid antibody status.
- Sick euthyroid syndrome—No treatment is needed. Repeat TSH after resolution of acute illness.

Management for Patients with Months of Life Expectancy

- Management is similar to patients with years of life expectancy. Thyroid replacement therapy is generally indicated

Management for Patients with Weeks/Days of Life Expectancy

- At the end of life patients may not be able to swallow. Replacement therapy with intravenous levothyroxine may be necessary, with a 0–50% dose reduction to adjust for oral bioavailability.
- Avoid frequent blood work if possible.

Recommended Reading

1. Lipman AJ, Lawrence DP. The management of fatigue in cancer patients. *Oncology* 2004;18(12):1527–1535.
2. Hui D. *Hypothyroidism in Approach to Internal Medicine (3rd ed.)*. Springer, New York, 2010.

Section IX

Rheumatology

Chapter 42

Arthritis

Maxine de la Cruz

Classification

There are approximately 200 types of arthritis that are generally split into three classes.

- Inflammatory arthritis
  - Rheumatoid arthritis (RA)
    - More common in women and affects several other parts of the body besides the joints
    - Can affect both large and small joints and those of the spine
  - Gout
    - Occurs with elevation of serum uric acid
    - Characterized by repeated episodes of pain and inflammation in more and more joints
  - Ankylosis spondylitis
    - Involves joints in the spine and sacroiliac joints
- Noninflammatory arthritis
  - Osteoarthritis
    - Results from overuse, trauma, or degeneration of joint cartilage as a result of aging
    - Occurs in weight-bearing joints such as the knee, hip, and spine and in joints used in work or sports such as the shoulder, wrists, hands, and elbows
  - Scoliosis
  - Posttraumatic arthritis
- Connective tissue disease
  - Lupus
    - Autoimmune disorder that affect joints, skin, brain, kidneys, and other organs
  - Sjogren's syndrome
    - Defined as dry eyes and mouth in the absence of other autoimmune disorders

Symptoms and Signs

- Symptoms—Joint pain, stiffness, weakness in the area affected

Table 42.1 Different Types of Arthritis and Associated Clinical Findings

Arthritis	Clinical Findings
Rheumatoid arthritis	Pleurisy, subcutaneous nodules
Gout	Fever, tophi around the affected joint
Ankylosis spondylitis	Fatigue, uveitis, anorexia, fever, weight loss
Lupus	Vary depending on organs affected at a given point in the disease: fatigue, fever, alopecia, rashes, light sensitivity, headaches, vision problems, abdominal pain, arrhythmias, mucositis
Sjogren's syndrome	Dry eyes and mouth, burning and itching of the eyes, loss of sense of taste, mouth sores, fever, difficulty swallowing or eating, thick saliva, hoarseness, fatigue

- Signs—Joint swelling, muscle atrophy near the affected joint (resulting from disuse), tenderness to palpation, limited range of motion, crepitus
- Other associated symptoms—Some types of arthritis can have clinical manifestations that are not related to the affected bony structures and the muscles that support them. Depending on the type of arthritis being considered in the differential diagnosis, other signs and symptoms may be present (Table 42.1).

Investigations

- A clinical history and careful physical examination are helpful in evaluating and identifying the type of arthritis the patient may have.
- Diagnostic tools include imaging studies of the involved joints [x-rays, ultrasound, and magnetic resonance imagings (MRIs)]. These are important to show the extent of damage to the joint.
- Serum markers that are specific to the type of arthritis being considered are also useful (Table 42.2).

Table 42.2 Different Types of Arthritis and Associated Laboratory Findings

Arthritis	Laboratory Findings
Rheumatoid arthritis	Complete blood count (CBC), C-reactive protein (CRP), erythrocyte sedimentation rate (ESR), rheumatoid factor, anti-CCP antibody, synovial fluid analysis
Gout	Synovial fluid analysis, serum uric acid, synovial biopsy, urinary uric acid
Ankylosis spondylitis	CBC, ESR, HLA-B27 antigen
Lupus	CBC, antinuclear antibody test, urinalysis to detect proteinuria, ESR
Sjogren's syndrome	Schirmer's test, antinuclear antibody test, salivary gland biopsy, slit lamp examination

Relevance to the Cancer Palliative Care Setting

- Biological agents place patients at increased risk of infections from bacteria, fungi, and viruses as well as development of some cancers such as leukemia and lymphoma in the long term.
- Acetaminophen and nonsteroidal antiinflammatory drugs (NSAIDs) may mask fever in cancer patients who are receiving chemotherapy, which is one of the key signs of febrile neutropenia. As a precautionary measure, cancer patients on chemotherapy should record their temperature each time before taking these analgesics.
- Careful assessment of pain syndromes must be done. Patients with no cancer-related pain should not be treated with opioids.
- Opioids that are used to treat cancer-related pain are also beneficial for symptomatic treatment of patients with arthritic pain. NSAIDs may be useful adjuvants to opioids in patients with arthritic pain.

Management for Patients with Years of Life Expectancy

- Several effective treatments for different types of arthritis can be used both to control the symptoms of pain that usually accompany such conditions as well as disease-modifying agents.
- However, caution must be taken as some of the drugs used can have serious side effects, particularly in patients receiving active cancer treatment.
- Analgesics are widely used for pain management and include NSAID agents that can cause gastrointestinal bleeding and cyclooxygenase (COX) 2-selective NSAIDs that reduce the gastrointestinal side effects seen with traditional NSAIDs but carry the risk of increased cardiac events in at-risk patients.
- Disease-modifying agents (methotrexate, leflunomide, sulfasalazine, hydroxychloroquine) that are used in rheumatoid arthritis may cause severe anemia.
- Treatment can also include corticosteroids and biological agents such as tumor necrosis factor (TNF) inhibitors, white blood cell modulators (rituximab and abatacept), and interleukin-6 (IL-6) inhibitors (tocilizumab) used to suppress the immune system thereby improving symptoms and slowing the progression of disease.
- Other complementary therapies are being investigated for use including nutritional supplements such as glucosamine (1,500 mg/day), chondroitin (800–1,200 mg/day), omega-3 supplements (12 g/day), gammalinolenic acid (1,400–2,800 mg/day), avocado/soybean unsaponafiables, and diacerein.
- Physical therapy and certain other forms of exercises can be used to decrease stiffness and strengthen muscles around the affected joints.
- Injections of cortisone and hyaluronic acid help to relieve pain and swelling and help in lubricating involved joints, respectively.

- Surgery may be considered if nonsurgical modalities have not provided pain relief and improved function.
- Dietary modifications are useful in reducing gouty attacks.

Management for Patients with Months of Life Expectancy

- Management is similar to patients with years of life expectancy.
- Optimization of function can be achieved by using agents to treat symptoms as they arise.

Management for Patients with Weeks/Days of Life Expectancy

- At the end of life, patients may not be able to swallow medications. If the patient is not symptomatic, then additional treatment with medications may not be appropriate.

Recommended Reading

1. Pirotta M. Arthritis disease—the use of complementary therapies. *Aust Fam Physician* 2010;39(9):638–640.
2. Sawitzke AD, et al. Clinical efficacy and safety of glucosamine, chondroitin sulphate, their combination, celecoxib or placebo taken to treat osteoarthritis of the knee: 2-year results from GAIT. *Ann Rheum Dis* 2010;69:1459.
3. Scott DL, Wolfe F, Huizinga TW. Rheumatoid arthritis. *Lancet* 2010;376 (9746):1094–1108.
4. Kruszka P, O'Brian RJ. Diagnosis and management of Sjogren syndrome. *Am Fam Physician* 2009;79:465–470.

Section X

Neuropsychiatric

Chapter 43

Acute Stroke Syndrome

Pedro Pérez-Cruz and Beatriz Shand

Classification

- Transient ischemic attack (TIA) and/or acute ischemic stroke (AIS)
  - Lacunar-lipohyalinosis
  - Thrombosis—Atherosclerotic, dissection, arteritis/vasculitis, fibromuscular dysplasia
  - Embolism—Atrial fibrillation, valvular heart disease, arrhythmia, endocarditis, patent foramen ovale
  - Hypoperfusion—Cardiac arrest, arrhythmia, massive pulmonary embolism, tamponade, bleeding
- Intracerebral hemorrhage (ICH)—Hypertension, brain tumors, trauma, bleeding diatheses, vasculitis, vascular malformations, aneurism rupture, amyloid angiopathy, illicit drugs (e.g., cocaine)
- Subarachnoid hemorrhage (SAH)—Trauma, aneurysm, vascular malformations, medications

Symptoms and Signs

- Symptoms—Acute onset of neurologic deficits, usually in seconds or minutes. Includes hemiplegia, numbness, diplopia, visual loss, dizziness, and speech disorders. Confusion may also be a presenting symptom.
- Signs—Pyramidal syndrome with flaccid paralysis at presentation, sensory impairment, ataxia, visual field defects, dysarthria, or aphasia.

Investigations

- Brain computed tomography (CT) scan without IV contrast is the first investigation to perform in the acute setting. This is a simple and fast test to discriminate between AIS, ICH, and SAH. It has diagnostic and prognostic implications. A clinical syndrome of acute neurologic deficit with a normal CT scan suggests AIS. Recovery of the neurologic deficit before 24 hours with a normal CT scan is compatible with a TIA. ICH is diagnosed when evidence of blood is seen in the cerebral parenchyma.
- Brain magnetic resonance imaging (MRI) is useful to diagnose AIS in a patient with a normal CT scan and to find specific etiologies of stroke. Angiography is useful in selected cases.

- Blood glucose and oxygenation can be used to rule out stroke mimics.
- Renal function and electrolytes may be useful to define treatment options and assess for complications such as hyponatremia. Complete blood count (CBC) and platelet count are useful to assess for thrombocytopenia. Prothrombin time (PT) and activated partial thromboplastin time (aPTT) can be used to assess coagulation. A lipid profile can detect hyperlipidemia as a risk factor for stroke.
- Electrocardiogram (EKG), cardiac enzymes, echocardiogram, carotid ultrasound, and continuous electrocardiography may be used to assess for possible etiologies and comorbidities. Etiologic studies should be performed to detect diseases for which useful and feasible interventions are available. The decision to study a particular patient should be made case by case.

Relevance to the Cancer Palliative Care Setting

- Cancer patients are at higher risk of developing AIS and ICH due to increased immobility (patent foramen ovale), cancer-related prothrombotic status, and medications (e.g., tamoxifen, bevacizumab, thalidomide).
- Acute stroke syndrome or complications such as delirium may impair the patient's ability to make decisions. If the patient is competent, assess his or her preferences and values with the presence of proxies.
- Consider brain metastases and tumor-related intracerebral hemorrhage in cancer patients presenting with acute neurologic deficits.
- Cancer patients may have increased risk of bleeding. Assess this risk in patients who are candidates for fibrinolytic therapy. In particular, brain metastases represent a contraindication for fibrinolytic therapy.
- Closely monitor depression and psychological symptoms as they might worsen functional outcomes and patient psychological distress.

Management for Patients with Years of Life Expectancy

- Prompt transfer to a certified stroke center is recommended when suspecting an acute stroke syndrome.
- Emergency room (ER) assessment: Complete medical and nurse evaluation with CT, blood samples, EKG, and evaluation by a neurologist.
- General supportive care: Oxygenation should be above 94%, sources of hyperthermia should be identified and treated with antipyretics, and hypovolemia and hypoglycemia/hyperglycemia should be monitored and corrected.
- Acute Ischemic Stroke
  - Fibrinolytic therapy: Consider the use of intravenous or intraarterial fibrinolysis according to the time from symptoms onset, patient medical and neurologic conditions, and therapy availability. Patients who receive fibrinolytic therapy have worse outcomes during the first 3-month

period postintervention. Benefits for neurologic outcomes are observed 3 months postintervention.
- Acute stroke unit admission to closely monitor and treat complications.
- Treat hypertension if blood pressure is higher than 220/120 mmHg.
- Aspirin 325 mg for all patients within 24 to 48 hours. The usefulness of clopidogrel and anticoagulants is not well established.
- No neuroprotective agents have shown improved outcomes.
- Acute neurologic complications should be monitored and assessed for all patients during the first days, particularly those with major infarctions.
- Intracerebral hemorrhage
  - Replacement of platelets or coagulation factors in patients with a severe coagulation factor deficiency or severe thrombocytopenia. Withhold oral anticoagulants and reverse anticoagulation if needed.
  - Initial monitoring and management should take place in an intensive care unit (ICU).
  - In regard to blood pressure control:
- If systolic blood pressure (SBP) >200 mmHg or mean arterial pressure (MAP) >150 mmHg consider aggressive treatment and monitoring.
- If SBP >180 mmHg or MAP >130 mmHg plus evidence of elevated intracranial pressure consider careful monitoring and treatment to keep cerebral perfusion pressure ≥60 mmHg.
- If SBP >180 mmHg or MAP >130 mmHg without evidence of elevated intracranial pressure consider careful monitoring and treatment to keep BP <160/90 mmHg or MAP <110 mmHg.
  - Neurosurgery evaluation is recommended for all patients.
- Patients with seizures should be treated with antiepileptic drugs.
  - Acute strokes may contribute to worsen patient functional status and independence. Rehabilitation should be initiated during admission.
  - Patients with TIAs and/or AIS have a 4–20% annual risk of a new ischemic event. Therefore, secondary prevention for cerebrovascular disease should be continued in patients with a long life expectancy.
- Smoking cessation and decreasing alcohol consumption in heavy drinkers should be recommended for all patients with TIAs or AIS.
- Aspirin—Evidence-based benefits for combined cardiovascular outcomes (stroke, acute myocardial infarction) are observed at 6 months of treatment. Benefits increase with longer treatment duration.
- Antihypertensives—Treatment of hypertension decreases the risk of new cardiovascular outcomes. Evidence-based benefits for combined cardiovascular outcomes are observed after 2 years of treatment.
- Statins—Decrease the risk of new cardiovascular outcomes (stroke and myocardial infarction). Benefits are observed after 3 years of treatment. Benefits increase with longer treatment duration.
- Carotid surgery—Decrease the risk of new strokes. Benefits are observed 2 years postintervention. It should not be recommended for patients with an estimated survival of less than 2 years. Carotid surgery is a high-risk procedure; therefore, assessment of risks and benefits for the particular patient is crucial.

Management for Patients with Months of Life Expectancy

- General management of acute stroke should be performed as above.
- Each treatment should be assessed weighing treatment-associated risks versus neurologic benefits. Carefully consider the time frame for expected benefits for each therapy.
  - Fibrinolytic therapy should not be used in patients with a life expectancy less than 3 months. Short-term bleeding risks are high and patients may not experience neurologic benefits.
  - Aspirin and statins may be recommended after balancing risks and benefits for the specific patient.
  - Carotid surgery should not be recommended in patients with only months of life expectancy.
- Modify treatments and interventions according to patient values and preferences.

Management for Patients with Weeks/Days of Life Expectancy

- The focus should be on symptom management and patient comfort.
- Transfer of a patient to an acute hospital should be discouraged given that interventions will not modify the patient´s medical and neurologic prognosis.
- Support family and proxies in decision making and in maintaining patient functioning and comfort.

Recommended Reading

1. Jauch EC, Saver JL, et al. Guidelines for the early management of patients with acute ischemic stroke: a guideline for healthcare professionals from the American Heart Association/American Stroke Association. *Stroke* 2013;44(3):870–947.

2. Morgenstern LB, Hemphill JC, et al. Guidelines for the management of spontaneous intracerebral hemorrhage: a guideline for healthcare professionals from the American Heart Association/American Stroke Association. *Stroke* 2010;41(9):2108–2129.

3. Vrecer M, Turk S, Drinovec J, Mrhar A. Use of statins in primary and secondary prevention of coronary heart disease and ischemic stroke. Meta-analysis of randomized trials. *Int J Clin Pharmacol Ther* 2003;41(12):567–577.

4. Sandercock PA, Counsell C, Gubitz GJ, Tseng MC. Antiplatelet therapy for acute ischaemic stroke. *Cochrane Database Syst Rev* 2008;(3):CD000029.

Chapter 44

Seizures

Ahsan Azhar, Ivo W. Tremont-Lukats, and Paul Walker

Classification

- Partial [arise from focal area of brain; the epileptogenic area can be readily identified on an electroencephalogram (EEG)]
  - Partial simple (no loss of consciousness); most partial seizures are motor, sensory, or both
  - Partial complex (alteration of consciousness)
- Generalized (most seizures in cancer patients begin as partial with secondary generalization. Propagation can be so fast that a partial onset is not evident clinically).
  - Absence seizures (patients stop what they are doing and have fixed, unresponsive gaze)
  - Tonic–clonic seizures (repetitive movements with rigidity alternating with rhythmic contractions/clonus; in lay terms known as *grand mal-type seizures*)

Symptoms and Signs

- Symptoms
  - Aura: These symptoms (which could be unpleasant but may also act as warning signals) precede the onset of generalized seizures and may include sensory (flashing of lights, sensation of pressure), autonomic (flushing, nausea, or palpitations), and/or affective (fear, anxiety déjà vu feelings, irritability) changes.
  - Generalized seizures may present as absence or tonic–clonic seizures (most common), tonic seizures (generalized muscle rigidity), clonic seizures (rhythmic contractions of muscle groups, mainly upper limbs, neck, and face), myoclonic seizures (brief segmental contractions of muscle groups; this type is common after brain anoxia from cardiac arrest), or atonic seizures (sudden, complete loss of muscle tone; not typically seen in cancer patients).
  - In the postictal phase (time period immediately following the seizure activity) the patients may exhibit somnolence, headaches, delirium, and new onset weakness mimicking a stroke (Todd paralysis or postictal hemiparesis).
  - Other symptoms include loss of consciousness or periods of "blackout" (no recollection of the event), tongue biting (nonspecific; patients with

severe syncope can also bite their tongues), fecal or urinary incontinence (nonspecific), and fall or trauma.

- Signs
  - Seizure activity depending upon the type of seizure.
  - Increased blood pressure and tachycardia may or may not be present.
  - Foaming at mouth (unable to swallow secretions, vomiting, with or without features of aspiration).
  - Absence or complex partial seizures may present as a staring gaze lasting about 5–10 seconds, along with associated stereotypical, purposeless movements such as lip smacking, repetitive blinking, fumbling, picking at clothes, and fidgeting.
  - Alteration or loss of consciousness (in complex partial and generalized seizures).
  - Deep cry or shouting (due to forced exhalation of air by sudden contraction of the diaphragm) seen mainly in primarily generalized tonic–clonic seizures.
  - Postictal phase might have features such as profuse sweating, prolonged sleep, and delirium.

Investigations

- Basic metabolic profile—Electrolytes, Ca, Mg, PO_4, blood urea nitrogen (BUN), creatinine (Cr), aspartate aminotransferase (AST), alanine aminotransferase (ALT), alkaline phosphatase (ALP), bilirubin, albumin, glucose level
- Brain imaging
- EEG

Relevance/Implications in Setting of Cancer Palliative Care

- Table 44.1 lists a number of common causes of seizures in cancer patients.
- Seizures potentiate the symptom burden, especially in terms of
  - Worsening the quality of life of a patient with advanced cancer.
  - Increased depression, fatigue, pain, and suffering, especially if recurrent or intractable.
  - Source of extreme distress for family and caregivers, especially if it is associated with trauma and bleeding (tongue bite, etc.) and may contribute to complicated grief.

Management of Status Epilepticus

- A traditional definition of status epilepticus was the continuous, uninterrupted seizure for more than 30 minutes. More common in cancer patients

Table 44.1 Common Causes of Seizures in Cancer Patients

Causes	Examples
Metabolic	Electrolyte disturbances (hypocalcemia, hyponatremia or hypernatremia, and hypoglycemia are the most frequent causes) Uremia of renal failure Hepatic encephalopathy
Neurologic	Primary brain tumors: all of them can cause seizures Metastasis to brain or meninges Encephalopathy (sepsis, any infection without sepsis, brain abscess) Cerebral vascular accidents (low platelets, platinum chemotherapy)
Drug toxicity	Chemotherapeutic agents (ifosfamide, methotrexate) High doses of opioids (especially in renal failure) Antipsychotics and tricyclic antidepressants (TCAs) (by reducing seizure threshold) Antibiotics (carbapenems, quinolones) Withdrawal (of opioids, benzodiazepines, alcohol)
Brain radiation	Very rare; however, patients with brain metastases or primary brain tumors can seize while receiving cranial irradiation

is the presence of several seizures of varying duration that do not let the patient recover before the next episode. This is known as *convulsive status epilepticus* or convulsive status.

- Many patients, especially those with a severe toxic-metabolic encephalopathy, enter into nonstop seizures. These seizures may not be obvious since there is no observable tonic–clonic activity; this is known as *nonepileptic status epilepticus* and can be confirmed only by EEG. It is a frequent complication in acutely ill bone marrow or stem cell transplant patients with hematologic malignancies and in the intensive care units.
- For convulsive status:
  - Ensure patient safety by protecting the airway and maintaining circulation.
  - Duration more than 5 minutes: Use a benzodiazepine such as lorazepam IV (1–2 mg at the rate of 2 mg/min; may repeat after 20 minutes) or midazolam IV (0.2 mg/kg as a bolus followed by a continuous IV infusion of 0.1–0.6 mg/kg/h. This may also be given subcutaneously. Other alternate routes are buccal or nasal—0.5 mg/kg). Midazolam is mostly used in the intensive care unit (ICU) setting.
  - Once seizures are controlled and the cause is treated, additional therapy may not be required; this is valid in cases of drug withdrawal, drug neurotoxicity, or seizures as part of the posterior encephalopathy syndrome (PRES). If maintenance therapy is started, acceptable choices are valproic acid (IV bolus 15 mg/kg over 15 minutes followed by continuous infusion at the rate of 1–2 mg/kg/h) or phenytoin (IV bolus 15–20 mg/kg over 30 minutes followed by 4–8 mg/kg/day in divided doses IV or PO). Fosphenytoin IV is safer than phenytoin in terms of hypotension and arrhythmias. Oral phenytoin should be given on an empty stomach to enhance absorption.
- Refractory status epilepticus (duration more than 60 minutes or no response to diazepam or lorazepam): May need to use palliative sedation with continuous midazolam infusion. In exceptional cases (based upon the

goals of care), anesthetic agents (such as propofol or pentobarbital) may be required along with sedation.

- If the cause of seizures is thought to be related to worsening brain edema, give adjuvant steroids (dexamethasone 4–6 mg IV q6h).

Management for Patients with Years of Life Expectancy

- General measures: Patients must be cautioned against driving or operating heavy machinery. They should be advised to wear a wrist band providing information about their condition and emergency contact information. The family should be educated on how to react in case of future seizures.
- Doses of commonly used anticonvulsant agents are given in Table 44.2.
- Conventional anticonvulsants have significant side effects as well as interactions. Newer agents are safer but lack intravenous formulations and require slow titrations.
- Blood levels of certain medications such as phenytoin need to be monitored; however, clinical response should guide the dosage.
- In postoperative cases of primary brain tumors, the antiseizure medication should be stopped 1 week after surgery.

Management of Patients with Months of Life Expectancy

- Management is similar to patients with years of life expectancy.
- Long-term prophylactic anticonvulsant therapy is generally not recommended in the palliative setting because of the potential for serious side effects and interactions these medications may pose.

Table 44.2 Common Dosages for Anticonvulsants

Anticonvulsant	Daily Dosage (Adults)
Carbamazepine	400–1,800 mg
Clobazam	10–30 mg
Gabapentin	1,800–3,600 mg
Lamotrigine	100–400 mg
Levetiracetam	500–4,000 mg
Oxcarbazepine	600–2,400 mg
Phenobarbital	1–5 mg/kg
Phenytoin	200–400 mg
Sodium valproate	1,000–3,000 mg
Pregabalin	150–600 mg
Topiramate	50–400 mg
Lacosamide	100–400 mg

- If the decision is made to stop anticonvulsants in an effort to simplify the medication list and to avoid side effects/interactions, these medications should be slowly tapered and never stopped abruptly.

Management for Patients with Weeks/Days of Life Expectancy

- Dysphagia may become an issue near the end of life. Conversion to a parenteral route is an option if access is available. Diazepam may be given as a suppository. Midazolam may also be given subcutaneously.
- Frequent blood work should be avoided.

Recommended Reading

1. Bruera E. *Textbook of Palliative Medicine*. Hodder Arnold, distributed by Oxford University Press, New York, 2006.

2. Hanks GWC. *Oxford Textbook of Palliative Medicine (4th ed.)*. Oxford University Press, New York, 2010: 1037–1042.

3. Gofton TE, Graber J, Carver A. Identifying the palliative care needs of patients living with cerebral tumors and metastases: a retrospective analysis. *J Neurooncol* [Research Support, Non-U.S. Gov't]. 2012;108(3):527–534.

4. Pace A, Villani V, Di Lorenzo C, et al. Epilepsy in the end-of-life phase in patients with high-grade gliomas. *J Neurooncol* 2013;111(1):83–86.

Chapter 45

Syncope

Jenny Wei

Classification

The causes of syncope can be divided into three general categories: neurally mediated, cardiac, and orthostatic.

Symptoms and Signs

- Syncope is a transient and abrupt loss of consciousness and postural tone associated with acute hypoperfusion of the bilateral cerebral hemispheres or the reticular activating system in the brainstem.
- It has a rapid onset followed by a complete and rapid recovery.
- Presyncopal symptoms such as dizziness, lightheadedness, weakness, fatigue, diaphoresis, and visual or auditory disturbances are common.
- Syncope may also occur without any warning symptoms.

Investigations

- The underlying etiology for syncope can often be identified from the initial evaluation. However, syncope can present various diagnostic challenges, as many episodes of transient loss of consciousness may occur as unwitnessed events with a limited available history.
- Many testing modalities are available in the evaluation of syncope. An electrocardiogram (EKG) plays an important role in the initial evaluation. The timing and order of investigation are guided by a thorough history and physical examination (see Table 45.1).

Relevance to the Cancer Palliative Care Setting

- Cancer patients are also at increased risk of falls secondary to old age, frailty, sarcopenia, and polypharmacy (e.g., benzodiazepine use). It is important to distinguish syncope (i.e., loss of consciousness) from accidental falls.
- In patients with advanced cancer autonomic dysfunction and dehydration may contribute to orthostatic hypotension leading to syncope.
- Cancer patients are also at risk of both embolic and hemorrhagic stroke (e.g., anticoagulants).

Table 45.1 Types of Syncope

Classification	Specific Etiologies	Examples	Diagnostic Tests to Consider	Treatment
Neurally mediated	Vasovagal syncope	Sight of blood, fear, pain, intense emotion	EKG Stress test and/or echocardiogram if risks for cardiac disease	Reassurance Lifestyle modifications
	Situational reflex syncope	Micturition, defecation, cough, sneezing, ocular pressure, swallow syncope	None Rule out cardiac disease if risk factors are present	Avoid triggering activity Lifestyle modifications
	Carotid sinus hypersensitivity	Neck movement, neck tumor, tight shirt collar	Carotid sinus massage Tilt table testing	Lifestyle modifications Consider cardiac pacing
Cardiac	Arrhythmias	Bradyarrhythmias or tachyarrhythmias	EKG, telemetry Holter monitoring, implantable loop recorder Electrophysiology study	Ablation therapy if indicated Implantable pacemakers Implantable cardioverter-defibrillator (ICD)
	Structural disease	Valvular disease, pump failure (ischemic cardiomyopathy), tamponade, myocardial infarction, pulmonary embolism, aortic dissection	Echocardiogram Stress test Cardiac catheterization if indicated EKG Cardiac biomarkers Computed tomography (CT) angiogram	Treat underlying mechanical/structural issue with surgical or medical management
Orthostatic	Drug induced	Diuretics, alcohol	Orthostatic challenge	Modification of medications
	Primary autonomic nervous system failure	Shy-Drager, Lewy body dementia	Orthostatic challenge Neurologic testing if indicated	Reverse underlying cause if possible Lifestyle modifications
	Secondary autonomic system failure	Diabetes, HIV, spinal cord injury, uremia, amyloid	Orthostatic challenge Neurologic testing to establish diagnosis if indicated	As above
	Volume depletion	Hemorrhage, diarrhea, emesis, venous pooling	Orthostatic challenge Volume challenge and retest	Volume repletion Compression stockings

Management for Patients with Years of Life Expectancy

• Management is dependent on the cause of syncope; see Table 45.1 for treatment guidelines.
• Hospitalization should be considered if a cardiac cause is suspected because cardiac syncope carries a worse prognosis than syncope that is neurally mediated or orthostatic in origin.
• In cancer patients with years of life expectancy management of syncope does not differ from patients without malignancy. For instance, in a cancer patient who has experienced a syncopal episode secondary to cardiac arrhythmia a full diagnostic workup and pacemaker implantation are appropriate.

Management for Patients with Months of Life Expectancy

• Diagnostic testing and management in these patients are similar to patients with years of life expectancy.

Management for Patient with Weeks/Days of Life Expectancy

• In patients with weeks of life expectancy, treatment may be similar to those for patients with years to months to years of life expectancy depending on the patient's overall functional status.
  • An appropriate approach should include a discussion about the goals of care with the patient and his or her family in this setting on a frequent basis, at least before and after diagnostic testing has been done.
  • Once the cause of syncope has been identified, a thorough consideration of the risks and benefits of all the treatment options should be exercised and discussed with the patient and his or her family.
• In patients with days of life expectancy, it may be appropriate to forgo aggressive testing and treatment as the benefits may be limited.

Recommended Reading

1. Freeman R. Syncope. In Longo DL, Fauci AS, Kasper DL, Hauser SL, Jameson JL, Loscalzo J (eds.). *Harrison's Principles of Internal Medicine* (18th ed.). McGraw-Hill, New York, 2012: Chapter 20. http://www.accessmedicine.com/content.aspx?aID=9095995. Accessed May 30, 2013.

2. Warrell DA, Firth JD, Cox TM (eds.). *Oxford Textbook of Medicine (5th ed.)*. Oxford University Press, New York, 2010.

3. Soteriades ES, Evans JC, Larson MG, et al. Incidence and prognosis of syncope. *N Engl J Med* 2002;347(12):878–885.

Chapter 46

Migraines

Jenny Wei

Classification

- Migraine without aura—Formerly referred to as "common migraine."
- Migraine with aura—Previously known as "classic migraine," associated with visual, auditory, taste, or smell disturbances 5–30 minutes prior to onset of headache.

Symptoms and Signs

- Symptoms—Table 46.1 lists the International Headache Society diagnostic criteria for migraine with and without aura. In general, migraines are episodic headaches lasting 4–72 hours. They are both more common and more severe in women than in men. Symptoms generally have an onset in adolescence or early adulthood. Table 46.2 lists the distinguishing features between migraine headaches and tension headaches.
- Signs—Migraines are characterized by benign and recurring headaches without specific signs.

Investigations

- The diagnosis of migraine is a clinical one. Imaging modalities or laboratory markers are not required for the diagnosis of migraine. Neuroimaging is generally not indicated for patients with migraine and normal neurologic examination. However, it is pertinent to differentiate migraines from secondary headaches in cancer patients as the presence of brain metastases, infection, and intracranial bleeding should be ruled out with laboratory studies and imaging modalities.
- Box 46.1 lists the alarming symptoms that should prompt consideration of neuroimaging.

Relevance to the Cancer Palliative Care Setting

- Migraine headaches are the second most common type of primary headaches affecting over 15% of women and 6% of men.

- Cancer patients may have concurrent migraines contributing to their overall symptom burden. This can lead to decreased functional status and poor quality of life.

Table 46.1 International Headache Society Diagnostic Criteria for Migraine with and without Aura

Migraine without aura

- At least five attacks with at least two of the following:
  Unilateral location
  Pulsating quality
  Moderate to severe pain intensity
  Aggravation with movement or causing avoidance of physical activity
- And one of the following symptoms during headache:
  Nausea or vomiting
  Photophobia or phonophobia
- Not attributed to another disorder

Migraine with aura

- Recurrent disorder manifesting in attacks of reversible focal neurologic symptoms that usually develop gradually over 5–20 minutes and last for less than 60 minutes
- Less commonly, headache lacks migrainous features or is completely absent
- Diagnostic criteria:
  Aura consisting of at least one of the following without motor weakness:
  - Fully reversible dysphasic speech disturbance
  - Sensory symptoms that are fully reversible, including positive features (pins and needles) and/or negative features (loss of vision)
  At least two of the following:
  - Homononymous visual symptoms and/or unilateral sensory symptoms
  - At least one aura symptom develops gradually over 5 minutes or different aura symptoms occur in succession over 5 minutes
  - Each symptom lasts at least 5 minutes, but no longer than 60 minutes
- Headaches fulfilling the criteria for migraine without aura begin during the aura or follow the aura within 60 minutes
- Not attributed to another disorder
- History of at least two attacks fulfilling the above criteria

Table 46.2 Distinguishing Features between Migraines and Tension Headaches		
Clinical Features	**Migraine Headaches**	**Tension Headaches**
Location	Unilateral	Bilateral
Quality	Pulsating	Nonpulsating
Intensity	Moderate to severe	Mild to moderate
Nausea/vomiting	Yes	No
Photophobia/ phonophobia	Yes	No
Aggravated by routine physical activity	Yes	No
Aura	Maybe	No

> **Box 46.1 Alarming Symptoms That Should Prompt Consideration of Neuroimaging**
>
> - Fever or other systemic symptoms
> - Focal neurologic signs or symptoms
> - Orbital bruit
> - Progressive worsening of headache despite appropriate therapy
> - Recent change in the pattern, frequency, or severity of headaches
> - Onset of headache with exertion, cough, or sexual activity
> - Onset of headache after age 40 years
> - Nocturnal occurrence or morning awakenings

Management of Patients with Years of Life Expectancy

- Nonsteroidal antiinflammatory drugs (NSAIDs)—Nonprescription NSAIDs can be used to reduce the severity and duration of acute migraine headaches (Table 46.3). NSAIDs are effective first-line drugs for mild to moderate migraine headaches and can be used in combination with acetaminophen, aspirin, and caffeine. The drug benefits are limited by bleeding risks, particularly in cancer patients receiving chemotherapy. Gastrointestinal, cardiac, and renal side effects are also limiting factors that should be considered prior to the initiation of NSAID therapy.

- 5-Hydroxytryptamine 1 (5-HT1) receptor agonists—Nonselective ergotamine and dihydroergotamine (DHE) may be used in selected patients, but the triptan drugs have largely replaced their use. The triptans are selective 5-HT1b/1d receptor agonists that are available in various formulations. All the triptan drugs are similar in their pharmacologic properties. Triptans are effective first-line therapies for moderate to severe migraine or mild to moderate migraine that has not responded to adequate doses of simple nonopioid analgesics. Side effects are usually mild and transient. They are not effective in migraines with aura unless given after aura is complete and headache has started. They do not always provide complete and rapid relief and often have to be combined with the use of an NSAID. Triptans and ergotamine are contraindicated in patients with cardiovascular or cerebrovascular disease.

- Dopamine antagonists—Metoclopramide, chlorpromazine, and prochlorperazine can be used as adjuvant therapy for relief of migraines. Metoclopramide can be used for associated nausea and delayed gastric emptying, which many cancer patients experience as a result of cancer treatment and/or the disease process.

- Dexamethasone—Used as adjunct therapy to abort acute migraines and may be a useful adjunct to standard therapy in preventing short-term headache recurrence. The long-term side effects limit its use, but it may be beneficial in decreasing overall symptom burden in cancer patients with shorter life expectancies (months to weeks/days).

Table 46.3 Dosages for Common Migraine Medications

Medications	Route/Dosing
• NSAIDs	
• Ibuprofen	• Oral: 200–800 mg q6–8h. Max: 2,400 mg/day
• Naproxen	• Oral: 250–500 mg q12h. Max: 1 g/day
• Ketorolac	• Oral: 10 mg q4–6h. Max: 40 mg/day
	• IV or IM: 15–30 mg × 1 q6h. Max: 120 mg/day; 60 mg/day if >65 years old or <50 kg
	• Duration of combined PO/IV/IM not to exceed 5 days; use the lowest effective dose and the shortest effective treatment duration
• Ergotamines	
• Dihydroergotamine	• IV or IM: 1 mg q1h × 2, up to 3 mg per attack, 6 mg/week
	• Intranasal (0.5 mg/spray): 1 spray in each nostril q15 min × 2, up to 4 sprays per attack, 6 sprays per day, 8 sprays per week
• Ergotamine 1 mg + caffeine 100 mg	• Oral: 1–2 tablets q30 min. Max: 6 mg ergotamine per day and 10 mg ergotamine per week
• Triptans	
• Sumatriptan	• Oral: 25–100 mg × 1, may repeat × 1 after 2 hours if headache recurs. Max: 200 mg/day. May follow initial 4–6 mg SC dose after 1 hour with 25–100 mg PO q2h × 1–2 doses, up to 100 mg PO per day
	• SC: 4–6 mg × 1, may repeat after 1 hour if headache recurs. Max: 12 mg/day
	• Intranasal (5 mg/spray, 20 mg/spray): 1 spray in one nostril × 1, may repeat q2h × 1 if headache recurs. Max: 40 mg/day
• Zolmitriptan	• Oral: 1.25–2.5 mg × 1, may repeat q2h × 1 if headache recurs. Max: 5 mg per episode, 10 mg/day
	• Oral disintegrating tablets: 2.5–5 mg × 1, may repeat × 1 after 2 hours. Max: 5 mg per episode, 10 mg/day
	• Intranasal: 1 spray (5 mg/spray) in one nostril × 1. May repeat q2h × 1 if headache recurs. Max: 2 sprays per day
• Rizatriptan	• Oral or oral disintegrating tablets: 5–10 mg × 1, may repeat dose q2h × 2. Max: 30 mg/day
• Naratriptan	• Oral: 1–2.5 mg × 1, may repeat q4h × 1 if partial response of headache recurs. Max: 5 mg/day
• Almotriptan	• Oral: 6.25–12.5mg × 1, may repeat dose q2h × 1 if headache recurs. Max: 25 mg/day
• Frovatriptan	• Oral: 2.5 mg × 1. May repeat dose × 1 q2h if headache recurs. Max: 7.5 mg/day
• Eletriptan	• Oral: 20–40 mg × 1. May repeat dose q2h × 1 if headache recurs. Max: 80 mg/day
• Dopamine antagonists	
• Metoclopramide	• Oral or IV or IM: 10 15 mg q6h
• Promethazine	• Oral or IV or IM: 12.5–25 mg q4–6h
• Prochlorperazine	• Oral or IV or IM: 5–10 mg q6–8h
• Dexamethasone	• IV: 10–25 mg, one time dose
• Other (combination drugs)	
• Acetaminophen 250 mg + aspirin 250 mg + caffeine 65 mg	• Oral: 2 tablets × 1. Max: 2 tablets per day, not to exceed 1 g in 4 hours and 4 g/day of acetaminophen, 4 g of aspirin per day from all sources

- Opioids—Generally reserved for the treatment of migraine headaches resistant to other therapies due to the potential for abuse and rebound headaches with long-term use.
- For patients with chronic migraine headaches (>15 headache episodes per month) with years of life expectancy consider the use of medications for migraine prophylaxis. Many patients can be managed adequately with low-dose anticonvulsants (topiramate, valproate, gabapentin), β-blockers (propranolol), or tricyclic antidepressants (TCAs; amitriptyline).

Management of Patients with Months of Life Expectancy

- Management is similar to patients with years of life expectancy.

Management of Patients with Weeks/Days of Life Expectancy

- Although the use of opioids for the treatment of migraines is generally not recommended, opioids may be appropriate for cancer patients with migraines at the end of life.
- Terminally ill cancer patients often have symptom burdens in excess of migraine alone; opioids can be used to concurrently palliate metastatic cancer pain and dyspnea. Prophylactic drugs may not be useful in this setting.

Recommended Reading

1. International Headache Society. HIS Classification ICHD-II. Migraine. http://his-classification.org/en/02_klassifikation/02_teil1/01.00.00_migraine.html. Accessed May 22, 2013.

2. Silberstein SD, Holland S, Freitag F, Dodick DW, Argoff C, Ashman E. Quality standards subcommittee of the American Academy of Neurology and the American Headache Society. Evidence-based guidelines update: Pharmacologic treatment for episodic migraine prevention in adults: report of the Quality Standards subcommittee of the American Academy of Neurology and the American Headache Society. *Neurology* 2012;78(17):1330–1345.

3. Gimore B, Michael M. Treatment of acute migraine headache. *Am Fam Physician* 2011;83(3):271–280.

4. International Headache Society. HIS Classification ICHD-II. Tension Type Headache. http://ihs-classification.org/en/02_klassifikation/02_teil1/02.01.00_tension.html. Accessed August 16, 2013.

Chapter 47

Neurocognitive Disorder (Dementia)

Wadih Rhondali and Marilene Filbet

Definition

- Dementia can be defined by progressive memory decline and at least one other cognitive domain (aphasia, apraxia, agnosia, or inability to perform executive function). The cognitive deficits should be severe enough to interfere with daily activities.
- In the latest update of the *Diagnostic and Statistical Manual of Mental Disorders* (*DSM-5*) dementia has been replaced by the terms "major and minor Neurocognitive Disorder." Table 47.1 lists the diagnostic criteria.

Causes

- Mild cognitive impairment (MCI; defined as a predementia state)
- Alzheimer's disease
- Vascular dementia
- Lewy body dementia
- Frontotemporal dementia
- Atypical dementia syndromes
- Parkinson's disease
- Traumatic brain injury
- Organic brain syndromes
- Pseudodementia

Symptoms

- Symptoms—Amnesia (memory impairment), aphasia (abnormal speech), apraxia (impaired performance of learned motor skills), agnosia (impaired recognition of people or objects), altered executive function (difficulty with planning, judgment, mental flexibility, abstraction, problem solving), behavioral disorders (distractibility, decline in personal hygiene), associated mood disorders (depression, anxiety). These deficits are characterized by gradual onset and continuing cognitive decline from a previous higher level of functioning.

Table 47.1 DSM-5 Diagnostic Criteria for Neurocognitive Disorders

Minor Neurocognitive Disorder	Major Neurocognitive Disorder	Delirium
• Evidence of modest cognitive decline in one or more of the cognitive domains (complex attention, executive function, learning and memory, language, perceptual-motor, social cognition) based on the concerns of the individual, a knowledgeable informant, or the clinician; and a decline in neurocognitive performance (i.e., between the 3rd and 16th percentiles) on formal testing. • The cognitive deficits are insufficient to interfere with independence. • Delirium excluded. • Other mental disorders (e.g., major depressive disorder, schizophrenia) excluded.	• Evidence of substantial cognitive decline in one or more of the cognitive domains based on the concerns of the individual, a knowledgeable informant, or the clinician; and a decline in neurocognitive performance (i.e., below the 3rd percentile) on formal testing. • The cognitive deficits are sufficient to interfere with independence. • Delirium excluded. • Other mental disorders (e.g., major depressive disorder, schizophrenia) excluded.	• Disturbance in attention (i.e., reduced ability to direct, focus, sustain, and shift attention) and orientation to the environment. • Disturbance develops over a short period of time (usually hours to a few days) and represents an acute change from baseline that is not solely attributable to another neurocognitive disorder and tends to fluctuate in severity during the course of a day. • A change in an additional cognitive domain, such as disorientation, memory deficit, or language disturbance, or a perceptual disturbance that is not better accounted for by a preexisting, established, or evolving other neurocognitive disorder; and • Disturbances must not occur in the context of a severely reduced level of arousal, such as coma.

Investigations

- Neuropsychological assessment starting with simple tests or screening instruments such as the Mini-Mental-State-Exam (MMSE).
- Brain imaging [brain magnetic resonance imaging (MRI) with coronal slices or brain computer tomography (CT) scan if unavailable] to eliminate secondary causes as subdural hematoma, chronic hydrocephalus, infection, brain tumor, or metastasis.
- Laboratory examinations can be used to assess potential causes of curable dementia. Typical tests include complete blood count (CBC) and differential, serum levels of urea, creatinine, free thyroxin (T_4), thyroid-stimulating hormone (TSH), albumin, liver enzymes, vitamin B_{12} and calcium, serology for syphilis, and in patients aged 60 years or younger, serology for HIV.

Relevance to the Cancer Palliative Care Setting

- Advanced dementia can complicate symptom assessment, patient–clinician communication, and complex decision making (e.g., cancer treatments and investigations, goals of care) and increase the risk of delirium.

- Cancer (e.g., brain tumors, brain metastases) and its treatments (e.g., whole brain irradiation, chemotherapy) can potentially result in cognitive impairment.
- During the last year of life, patients with dementia often experience confusion (83%), urinary incontinence (72%), pain (64%), low mood (61%), constipation (59%), and loss of appetite (57%). These symptoms are similar to those that typically occur in patients with advanced cancer in the last few weeks of life.

Management for Patients with Years of Life Expectancy

- Palliative care for patients with incurable dementia (e.g., Alzheimer's disease, dementia with Lewy bodies) should be offered in conjunction with appropriate medical treatments starting at the time of diagnosis. Early referral to palliative care can help caregivers discuss and document advanced directives with patients at earlier stages of dementia and can provide longitudinal support to caregivers during the trajectory of the illness. Some of the commonly used treatments are listed below:
- Acetylcholinesterase inhibitors (donepezil and galantamine)—Can be used for mild cognitive impairment, mild-to-moderate Alzheimer's disease, and Lewy body dementia.
- N-Methyl-D-aspartate (NMDA) antagonist (memantine)—Can be combined with acetylcholinesterase inhibitors in mild-to-moderate Alzheimer's disease in case of inadequate response to monotherapy and in severe Alzheimer's disease.
- Control of hypertension and diabetes—First-line treatment for mild to moderate vascular or mixed dementia.
- Antipsychotics—Often used to treat disruptive behavior, agitation, and aggression but they are not usually recommended for treating dementia. Prefer atypical antipsychotics.
- Psychological treatments—Do not slow down dementia progression but can help to cope with the illness and its symptoms (e.g., maintenance cognitive stimulation therapy).

Management for Patients with Months of Life Expectancy

- Management is similar to patients with years of life expectancy with less aggressive treatment for dementia and a switch toward patient's quality of life and comfort.

Management for Patients with Weeks/Days of Life Expectancy

- Patients with advanced dementia suffer a range of symptoms similar to those found in advanced cancer patients (e.g., pain, dyspnea, pressure sores, agitation, difficulty swallowing, and loss of appetite).

• At the end of life patients may not be able to swallow. Symptomatic treatments should be administered subcutaneously or intravenously.

• The use of tube feeding in patients with advanced dementia is not recommended.

Recommended Reading

1. Alexopoulos GS, Jeste DV, Chung H, Carpenter D, Ross R, Docherty JP. The expert consensus guideline series. Treatment of dementia and its behavioral disturbances. Introduction: methods, commentary, and summary. *Postgrad Med* 2005;Spec No:6–22.

2. Hughes JC, Jolley D, Jordan A, Sampson EL. Palliative care in dementia: issues and evidence. *Adv Psychiatr Treat* 2007;13(4):251–260.

3. McCarthy M, Addington-Hall J, Altmann D. The experience of dying with dementia: a retrospective study. *Int J Geriatr Psychiatr* 1997;12(3):404–409.

Chapter 48

Vitamin B$_{12}$ Deficiency

Maxine de la Cruz

Pathophysiology

- Vitamin B$_{12}$ (cobalamin) is essential in DNA synthesis and cellular metabolism. It is vital in the development and initial myelination of the central nervous system and maintenance of normal function.
- Vitamin B$_{12}$ metabolism is complex and defects in any of the stages of metabolism can result in clinically significant deficiency.
  - 1–5% of free cobalamin is absorbed along the gastrointestinal tract by diffusion.
  - Vitamin B is a cofactor for methionine synthase and L-methylmalonyl-coenzyme A (CoA) mutase. Methionine synthase is essential for purine and pyrimidine synthesis. Failure of this process results in the development of megaloblastic anemia. L-Methylmalonyl-CoA mutase converts methylmalonyl CoA to succinyl CoA. Deficiency of vitamin B$_{12}$ leads to accumulation of methylmalonyl CoA that is thought to be responsible for the neurologic symptoms observed.
- The presence of dyssynchrony between the maturation of the cytoplasm and the nucleus results in macrocytosis, immature nuclei, and hypersegmentation in granulocytes. Ineffective erythropoiesis causes intramedullary hemolysis.
- Vitamin B$_{12}$ deficiency is a reversible cause of bone marrow failure (megaloblastic anemia) and demyelinating disease of the nervous system.
- 50–90% of cobalamin stores in the body (3–5 mg) are located in the liver and delay clinical manifestation of deficiency for up to 5 years.
- Diseases associated with vitamin B$_{12}$ deficiency include thyroid disease, vitiligo, diabetes mellitus, iron deficiency, osteoporosis, dementia, age-related macular degeneration, and depression.

Causes

- Gastric
  - Food-cobalamin malabsorption—Atrophic gastritis, chronic gastritis, protein-bound vitamin B$_{12}$ malabsorption
- Autoimmune—Pernicious anemia (autoimmune gastritis), scleroderma, Sjogren's syndrome
- Surgery—Total or partial gastrectomy, gastric bypass or other bariatric surgery, ileal resection

- Intestinal malabsorption—Inflammatory bowel disease, Imerslund–Grasbeck and other syndromes, intestinal lymphomas, bacterial overgrowth, amyloidosis
- Drugs—Metformin, PPI, H2 blockers, antacids, colchicine, nitrous oxide
- Dietary deficiency—Vegan or vegetarian diet, diets low in meat and dairy, alcoholism

Symptoms and Signs

- Symptoms—Fatigue, pallor, fast or irregular heartbeat, dizziness, dyspnea, cognitive problems, cold extremities, weakness, headache, depression, mania, hallucinations, symmetric paresthesias, and gait abnormalities
- Signs—Pallor, hyperpigmentation, jaundice, edema, glossitis, malabsorption, infertility and thrombosis, impaired vibration sense and proprioception, ataxia, abnormal reflexes, orthostatic hypotension, and optic atrophy

Investigations

- Serum vitamin B_{12} level is the first test to confirm a diagnosis of vitamin B_{12} deficiency. Establish that a normal serum vitamin B level is 180–900 pg/ml.
- Measurement of methylmalonic acid (MMA) and homocysteine (Hcy) levels if serum levels are below 350 pg/ml. MMA and Hcy are elevated in the majority of patients with clinical vitamin B_{12} deficiency. Normal levels of MMA and Hcy suggest the absence of vitamin B_{12} deficiency.
- Bone marrow aspiration and biopsy are unnecessary and results can be mistaken for acute leukemia.

Relevance to the Cancer Palliative Care Setting

- Vitamin B_{12} deficiency is common in the elderly (40%).
- Vitamin B_{12} deficiency can occur in patients with gastrointestinal (GI) surgeries as a result of either the cancer or complications from its treatment.
- Drugs can also reduce the absorption of vitamin B_{12} from the GI tract.
- Deficiency in vitamin B_{12} contributes to symptom burden and may be overlooked as a possible etiology in those with fatigue, weakness, even depression, paresthesias, ataxia, and delirium in severe cases.

Management for Patients with Years of Life Expectancy

- Vitamin B_{12} replacement—The classic treatment of vitamin B_{12} deficiency is parenteral administration of vitamin B_{12}. Other routes include intramuscular injections as well as oral and nasal administration. It is given primarily in the form of cyanocobalamin, or hydroxycobalamin, or methylcobalamin. The dose range is from 100 to 1,000 µg/month (or every 2–3 months when hydroxycobalamin is given).

- Oral doses of 1,000–2,000 µg/day have likewise been used to induce and maintain remission in patients with megaloblastic anemia. But evidence is lacking for those patients with more severe neurologic manifestations.

- Transnasal and buccal preparations are also available.

- Obtain repeat levels of serum vitamin B$_{12}$, MMSA, and Hcy levels in 4–6 weeks of treatment to assess the response. Once mid-normal levels are achieved, monitor levels every 6–12 months.

Management for Patients with Months of Life Expectancy

- Management is similar to patients with years of life expectancy. Usually the oral route is preferred as it is more convenient for the patient.

Management for Patients with Weeks/Days of Life Expectancy

- There is no set guideline for treatment at the end of life. It is reasonable to forego replacement in patients with very limited life expectancies.

- Patients may not be able to swallow pills and administration via the intramuscular route may result in more discomfort.

- Resulting symptoms of vitamin B$_{12}$ deficiency may also be treated with other agents if necessary.

- Symptom burdens often have multiple etiologies that normalization of vitamin B$_{12}$ levels alone may not be sufficient to reverse.

Recommended Reading

1. O'Leary F, Samman S. Vitamin B12 in health and disease. *Nutrients* 2010;2(3): 299–316.

2. Stabler SP. Clinical practice. Vitamin B12 deficiency. *N Engl J Med* 2013;368(2):149–160.

3. Lachner C, Steinle NI, Regenold WT. The neuropsychiatry of vitamin B12 deficiency in elderly patients. *J Neuropsychiat Clin Neurosci* 2012;24(1):5–15.

4. Andres E, Fothergill H, Mecili M. Efficacy of oral cobalamin (vitamin B12) therapy. *Expert Opin Pharmacother* 2010;11(2):249–256.

Chapter 49

Parkinson's Disease

Shobha Rao

Causes

- Idiopathic Parkinson's disease (PD)—No specific identifiable cause.
- Mutations in parkin gene—Important in early-onset PD.
- Other risk factors include head injury, pesticide exposure, use of hypnotic, anxiolytic, or antidepressant for >1 year, and family history of Parkinson's disease.

Symptoms and Signs

- Motor symptoms include rigidity, tremors, bradykinesia, difficulty getting out of chair, opening jars, difficulty turning in bed, change in handwriting (micrographia), loss of balance, and shuffling gait.
- Nonmotor manifestations of PD are listed in Table 49.1 and include various sleep, neuropsychiatric, gastrointestinal, and autonomic symptoms.

Investigations

- Diagnosis of PD is clinical and requires the presence of bradykinesia plus rigidity or tremor.
- Asymmetrical onset of symptoms and clinical improvement with levodopa are supportive of the diagnosis.
- Perform computed tomography (CT) or a magnetic resonance imaging (MRI) when the diagnosis of PD is uncertain to rule out other causes of parkinsonisms such as vascular problems, tumor, normal-pressure hydrocephalus, and progressive supranuclear palsy.

Relevance to the Cancer Palliative Care Setting

- Levodopa is listed as "contraindicated" in patients with malignant melanoma in the prescribing literature. Although patients with PD are at increased risk for developing malignant melanoma, evidence does not suggest a causal relationship between levodopa therapy and exacerbation of malignant melanoma.

Table 49.1 Management of Nonmotor Symptoms

Symptoms		Management
Sleep problems	Nocturia, anxiety/depression	Sleep hygiene, diagnose and treat anxiety/depression
	Nocturnal rigidity, dystonia	Extended release carbidopa/levodopa
	OSA	CPAP
	RLS	Dopamine agonist or levodopa
	REM sleep behavior disorder	Clonazepam
	Excessive daytime sleepiness	Adjust dose if on DA, modafinil
Neuropsychiatric	Depression/anxiety	SSRI (favorable side effect profile), nortriptyline and desipramine, SSRI and benzodiazepines for anxiety
	Fatigue/apathy	Optimize treatment for depression, methylphenidate
	Psychosis	Treat reversible causes—infection, metabolic disturbances, side effects of medications Cholinesterase inhibitors for dementia Quetiapine, clozapine (may cause agranulocytosis)
	Dementia	Cholinesterase inhibitors–rivastigmine, FDA approved for dementia in PD
	Delirium	Reversible causes—infection, dehydration, and electrolyte abnormalities, decrease or discontinue anticholinergics, MAO-B inhibitors, amantadine, and dopamine agonists May use quetiapine
Pain	Musculoskeletal, neuropathic, psychosocial	Careful adjustment of antiparkinsonian medications, judicious use of opioids, and adjuvant therapy (e.g., gabapentin, TCA for neuropathic pain), antidepressants
Gastrointestinal	Dysphagia	Speech pathology referral, safe swallowing techniques, dietary modification, adjust PD medicines (dysphagia improves in "on" phase)
	Constipation	Dietary modification, stool softeners and laxatives, tegaserod, domperidone, polyethylene glycol
Autonomic	Drooling	Botulinum toxin A (Botox), glycopyrrolate
	Orthostatic hypotension	Increase salt and fluid intake, compression stockings
	Urinary symptoms	Rule out bladder infection, reduce evening fluid intake, timed voiding, oxybutynin and tolterodine, solifenacin, and darifenacin

Abbreviations: CPAP, continuous positive airway pressure; DA, dopamine agonist; FDA, Food and Drug Administration; PD, Parkinson's disease; REM, rapid eye movement; RLS, restless leg syndrome; SSRI, selective serotonin reuptake inhibitors; TCA, tricyclic antidepressant; OSA, obstructive sleep apnea.

Modified from Kelvin L, Chou MD. Parkinson disease. *Ann Intern Med* 2012;157(9):ITC5-1.

- Metoclopramide and phenothiazines are commonly used in cancer patients for palliation of symptoms. These medications can cause marked extrapyramidal symptoms (EPS) in people with PD. Domperidone can be used to treat gastrointestinal symptoms as it does not cross the blood–brain barrier and is less likely to cause EPS. However, domperidone is not FDA approved. It is available in Canada and the United Kingdom but not in the United States.
- Quetiapine (Seroquel) is usually prescribed for managing delirium in PD patients because it is less likely to cause extrapyramidal symptoms.
- Symptoms such as constipation, cachexia, nausea/vomiting, and delirium can add to the symptom burden in PD patients with cancer.

Management of Patients with Years of Life Expectancy

- Dopaminergic therapy with either carbidopa/levodopa or a dopamine agonist (e.g., pramipexole, ropinirole, rotigotine) should be initiated to control motor symptoms (see Table 49.2).
- Carbidopa/levodopa (Sinemet) is the most effective agent for treatment of PD. However, long-term use (>5 years) is associated with the development of motor complications such as dyskinesias and "wearing off" (shorter duration of benefit with each levodopa dose). For patients who develop dyskinesia, reducing the dose of levodopa and adding a DA or amantadine are helpful.
- Strategies to treat "wearing off" include adding a dopamine agonist, increasing the levodopa dosage and frequency, starting a catechol-O-methyl transferase inhibitor such as entacapone, or adding a monoamine oxidase B (MAO-B) inhibitor (e.g., selegiline, rasagiline).
- Consider referral for deep-brain stimulation for advanced disease with severe motor fluctuations, dyskinesia, or disabling tremors that are not responding to adequate drug therapy.
- See Table 49.1 for the management of nonmotor symptoms of PD.
- Pain may be a problem in all stages of PD. Pain can be due to musculoskeletal, neuropathic, or psychosocial causes. Successful pain management strategies include evaluation of the type of pain, careful adjustment of antiparkinsonian medications, judicious use of pain medications, and adjuvant therapy as needed. Side effects of opiates can be exacerbated due to coexisting constipation and gastroparesis in patients with PD.
- Initiate goals of care discussion regarding PEG tube and code status early.

Management of patients with Months of Life Expectancy

- Management of motor and nonmotor symptoms is similar to patients with years of life expectancy.

Table 49.2 Typical Medications and Doses for Parkinson's Disease

Class	Common Medications/ Available Doses in mg	Dose
Carbidopa/ levodopa	Carbidopa/levodopa (Sinemet) 10/100, 25/100, 50/200	25/100 mg 2–3 times/day
Carbidopa/ levodopa (controlled release)	Carbidopa/levodopa (controlled release) (Sinemet CR) 10/100, 25/100, 50/200	50/200 mg 2 times/day
Dopamine agonist	Pramipexole (Mirapex) 0.125, 0.25, 0.5, 1.0, 1.5	2 to 6 times a day for a maximum dose 4.5 mg/day
	Ropinirole (Requip) 0.25, 0.5, 1, 2, 3, 4, 5	2 to 6 times a day for a maximum dose of 24 mg/day
	Rotigotine transdermal system (Neupro®) 2 mg/24 h, 4 mg/24 h, 6 mg/24 h, 8 mg/24 h	One 2 mg patch per day
Anticholinergics	Benzotropine mesylate (Cogentin) 0.5	0.5 mg 2 times/day
	Trihexyphenidyl (Artane) 1, 2	1–2 mg 2 times/day
MAO-B inhibitors	Selegiline 5 mg	5 mg 2 times/day
	Rasagiline 0.5, 1	0.5 mg once daily
COMT inhibitors	Entacapone (Comtan) 200	200 mg with levodopa Maximum dose 8 mg/day
	Tolcapne (Tasmar) 100, 200	100 mg 3 times/day
NMDA antagonist	Amantadine (Symmetral) 100 mg	100 mg 2 to 3 times/day
Cholinesterase inhibitors	Rivastigmine 1.5, 3, 4.5, 6 Patch 10, 20	1.5 mg 2 times/day Patch 10 (9.5 mg/24 h) Patch 20 (17.4 mg/24 h)

Abbreviations: MAO-B inhibitors, monoamine oxidase B inhibitors; COMT inhibitors, catechol-O-methyltransferase inhibitors, NMDA antagonist, N-methyl-D-aspartate receptor.

- Nonmotor symptoms such as dementia, depression, psychosis, and autonomic dysfunction predominate.
- Evaluate for caregiver stress as patients develop significant physical disability and cognitive decline.

Management of Patients with Weeks/Days of Life Expectancy

- Patients often develop worsening of swallowing problems.
- Dietary modification such as honey thickened fluids is helpful to increase feeding efficiency and reduce the risk of aspiration.

- If unable to take medicines by mouth transdermal, rectal, or subcutaneous use of medications may be necessary.
- Management should focus on a supportive and palliative approach to control symptoms (see Table 49.1 for symptom management).

Recommended Reading

1. Scott WK, Nance MA, et al. Complete genomic screen in Parkinson disease: evidence for multiple genes. *JAMA* 2001;286(18):2239–2244.

2. Rao G, Fisch L, Srinivasan S, et al. Does this patient have Parkinson disease? *JAMA* 2003;289(3):347–353.

3. Kelvin L, Chou MD. Parkinson disease. *Ann Intern Med* 2012;157(9):ITC5-1.

Index

Page numbers in **bold** indicate material that is the subject of a chapter. Page numbers followed by *t* or *f* indicate a table or figure on the designated page.